Nurse Prescribers' Formulary
for Community Practitioners

NPF 2013 2015

BMA PHARMACEUTICAL SOCIETY

Published jointly by
BMJ Group
Tavistock Square, London WC1H 9JP, UK
and
Pharmaceutical Press
Pharmaceutical Press is the publishing division of the
Royal Pharmaceutical Society
1 Lambeth High Street, London, SE1 7JN, UK

ISBN: 978 0 85711 125 8

ISSN: 1468-4853

Printed by Advent Colour, Andover, UK

Typeset by Data Standards Ltd

**Copies may be obtained through any bookseller or
direct from:**

Pharmaceutical Press
c/o Macmillan Distribution (MDL)
Brunel Rd
Houndmills
Basingstoke
RG21 6XS
UK
Tel: +44 (0) 1256 302 699
Fax: +44 (0) 1256 812 521
E-mail: direct@macmillan.co.uk
www.pharmpress.com

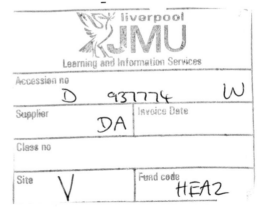

Preface

The Nurse Prescribers' Formulary for Community Practitioners (formerly the Nurse Prescribers' Formulary for District Nurses and Health Visitors) is for use by District Nurses and Specialist Community Public Health Nurses (including Health Visitors) who have received nurse prescriber training. It provides details of preparations that can be prescribed for patients receiving NHS treatment on form FP10P (form HS21(N) in Northern Ireland, form GP10(N) in Scotland, forms WP10CN and WP10PN in Wales).

Community Practitioner nurse prescribers should prescribe only from the list of preparations in the Nurse Prescribers' Formulary for Community Practitioners (for conditions specified in the NPF). Most medicinal preparations should be prescribed by generic titles as shown under the individual monographs in the NPF; however, some medicinal preparations and a majority of appliances may need to be prescribed by brand name—see individual product entries in the NPF.

The Nurse Prescribers' Advisory Group (formerly the Nurse Prescribers' Formulary Subcommittee) (p. iv) oversees the preparation of the NPF for Community Practitioners and advises the UK health ministers on the list of preparations that may be prescribed by Community Practitioner nurse prescribers.

The list of preparations from which Community Practitioner nurse prescribers may prescribe is reviewed constantly in the light of comments from nurse prescribers and applications from manufacturers.

The NPF has been designed for use with the British National Formulary (BNF); it forms an appendix to the BNF and as such is termed the Nurse Prescribers' Formulary Appendix (Appendix NPF). The current edition of the NPF includes Appendix 5 (Wound Management Products and Elasticated Garments) from BNF 66 (September 2013).

The Nurse Prescribers' Advisory Group records its thanks to BNF staff for their help with the preparation of this edition. F. Gibson and staff provided valuable technical assistance. Data Standards Ltd have provided assistance with typesetting.

The Nurse Prescribers' Advisory Group is grateful to those who have commented on previous editions of the NPF. In order that future editions of the NPF for Community Practitioners are able to reflect the requirements of nurse prescribers, users are urged to send comments and constructive criticism to:

NPF/BNF,
Royal Pharmaceutical Society
1 Lambeth High Street, London SE1 7JN.
editor@bnf.org

Contents

This edition of the NPF is intended as a pocket book for rapid reference and so cannot contain all the information necessary for patient management. For additional information the nurse prescriber should refer to the BNF or to the doctor who will have access to further information including manufacturers' product literature. Supplementary information is also available from pharmacists. Information is also available from medicines information services (see inside front cover).

Nurse Prescribers' Advisory Group 2013

Chair
Molly Courtenay
PhD, MSc, Cert Ed, BSc, RGN

Committee Members
Duncan S.T. Enright
MA, PGCE, MInstP

Penny M. Franklin
RN, RCN, RSCPHN(HV), MA, PGCE

Belén Granell Villén
BSc, PGDipClinPharm

Tracy Hall
BSc, MSc, RGN, DN, Dip N, Cert N

Margaret F. Helliwell
MB, BS, BSc, MFPHM FRCP (Edin), MRCGP

Jill Hill
RGN, BSc

Bryony Jordan
BSc, DipPharmPract, MRPharmS

Suhas Khanderia
BPharm, MSc, MBA, MRPharmS

Sandra Lawton
RN, RN Dip (Child), ENB 393, MSc

Joan Myers
OBE, MSc, BSc, RGN, RSCN, Dip DN

Wendy J. Nicholson
BSc, MA, Cert Ed, RGN, RSCN

Jill M. Shearer
BSc, RGN, RM

Vicky Vidler
MA, RGN, RSCN

John Wright

Executive Secretary
Heidi Homar
BA

Nurse Prescribers' Formulary for Community Practitioners

Prescription Writing

Further information may be found in BNF pp. 1–6

Prescriptions written by nurse prescribers should:

- be computer printed or written legibly in ink;
- be dated;
- state patient's full name and address;
- be signed in ink by the prescriber;
- include age and date of birth of patient.

Also recommended:

- Dose and the dose frequency should be stated. For preparations to be taken 'as required' **a minimum dose interval** should be specified, e.g. 'every 4 hours'.
- The unnecessary use of decimal points should be avoided, e.g. 3 mg, not 3.0 mg.
- Strength of the preparation should be stated, e.g. Paracetamol Tablets 500 mg.
- Quantities of 1 gram or more should be written as 1 g etc.
- Quantities of less than 1 gram should be written in milligrams, e.g. 500 mg, not 0.5 g (see inside back cover of BNF for conversion guide). It is, however, acceptable to express a range in the decimal form, e.g. 0.5 to 1 g.
- Quantity prescribed should generally be the pack size specified in the NPF under each preparation.
- Names of medicines should be written clearly using approved (generic) titles or proprietary names as specified throughout the NPF and should **not** be abbreviated.
- Directions should be in **English** and should not be abbreviated.

Security and validity of prescriptions

In order to ensure the security and validity of prescriptions nurse prescribers should:

- not leave them unattended;
- not leave them in a car where they may be visible;
- keep them locked up when not in use.

When there is any doubt about the authenticity of a prescription, the pharmacist will contact the nurse prescriber; see also Incomplete Prescriptions, below.

Children

Prescriptions should be written according to the guidelines above, stating the child's age.

Children's doses are stated in the NPF where appropriate but nurse prescribers should prescribe for children only if it is within their competence and after a full assessment (bearing in mind the differences in assessment between adults and children).

Where a single dose is stated for a given age range, it applies to the middle of the age range and may need to be adjusted to obtain doses for ages at the lower and upper limits of the stated range. Nurse prescribers are advised to err on the side of caution.

The pharmacist will supply an **oral syringe** with oral liquid preparations if the dose prescribed is less than 5 mL. The oral syringe is marked in 0.5-mL divisions from 1 to 5 mL to measure doses of less than 5 mL (other sizes of oral syringe may also be available). It is provided with an adaptor and an instruction leaflet. A 5-mL spoon will be given for doses of 5 or 10 mL.

> For detailed advice on medicines for children consult *BNF for Children.*

Unlicensed and 'off-label' prescribing

In general the *doses, indications, cautions, contra-indications*, and *side-effects* in the NPF reflect those in the manufacturers' data sheets or Summaries of Product Characteristics (SPCs) which, in turn, reflect those in the corresponding marketing authorisations or product licences.

Community Practitioner Nurse Prescribers should not prescribe unlicensed medicines, that is, medicines without a valid marketing authorisation or product licence. Neither should they prescribe licensed medicines for uses, doses, or routes that are outside the product licence (unlicensed use, 'off-label' use, or 'off-licence' use). The only exception is nystatin which may be prescribed for neonates under certain circumstances (see p. 18).

Excipients

Where an oral liquid medicine in the NPF is available in a form free of *fructose, glucose,* or *sucrose* a note has been added to say that a sugar-free version may be requested by adding 'sugar free' to the prescription. Preparations containing hydrogenated glucose syrup, mannitol, maltitol, sorbitol, or xylitol are also marked 'sugar-free' because there is evidence that they do not cause dental caries. Whenever possible sugar-free preparations should be requested for children to reduce the risk of dental decay.

Where information on the presence of *aspartame, gluten, tartrazine, arachis (peanut) oil* or *sesame oil* is available, this is indicated against the relevant product entry; in the absence of information on excipients in the NPF or in the product literature, then the manufacturer should be contacted.

Information is provided on *selected excipients* in skin preparations (see BNF section 13.1.3).

Prevention of adverse reactions

Adverse reactions may be prevented as follows:

- Never prescribe any medicine unless there is a good indication.

- A Community Practitioner nurse prescriber should **not** prescribe medicines for pregnant women (except folic acid and, in some circumstances, nicotine replacement therapy); the patient should be referred to her doctor.

- It is very important to recognise allergy as a cause of adverse drug reactions. Ask if the patient has had any previous reactions, particularly when prescribing aspirin or dressings impregnated with iodine.

- Ask if the patient is taking any other medicines **including self medication**; remember that aspirin interacts with warfarin.

- Check whether there are any special instructions in relation to hepatic or renal disease.

- Prescribe as few medicines as possible and give very clear instructions to the elderly or any patient likely to misunderstand complicated instructions. Elderly patients cannot normally cope with more than three different medicines (and ideally they should not need to be taken more than twice daily).

Reporting of adverse reactions

If a patient has a suspected adverse reaction to a medicine or dressing, the nurse prescriber should consider reporting it to the Medicines and Healthcare products Regulatory Agency (MHRA) through the Yellow Card Scheme for reporting adverse reactions.

Yellow Cards for reporting are bound in this book (inside back cover); alternatively, an electronic form is available at yellowcard.mhra.gov.uk.

For more details on adverse reactions to drugs and on reporting, see BNF p.12.

Incomplete prescriptions

A pharmacist may need to contact the nurse prescriber if the *quantity, strength* or *dose* are missing from the prescription. The pharmacist will then arrange for the missing details to be added. Under some circumstances the pharmacist will use professional judgement as to what to give and will endorse the prescription.

Labelling of dispensed medicine

The following will appear on the label of a dispensed medicine:

- name of product
- name of patient
- date of dispensing
- name and address of pharmacy
- directions for use
- total quantity of product dispensed
- advice to keep out of reach of children.

Other information (e.g. 'flammable') will be added by the pharmacist as appropriate. Preparation entries in the NPF provide details of any additional cautionary advice that the pharmacist will add.

The *name of the product* will be that which is written on the prescription.

Safety in the home

Patients must be warned to keep all medicines out of the reach of children. Medicines will be dispensed in reclosable *child-resistant containers* unless:

- they are in manufacturers' original packs designed for supplying to the patient
- the patient would have difficulty in opening a child-resistant container.

In the latter case the pharmacist will make a particular point of advising that the medicines be kept out of reach of children. The nurse prescriber could usefully *reinforce this advice*.

Patients should be advised to dispose of *unwanted medicines* by returning them to a pharmacist for destruction.

Duplicate medicines

Nurses are well placed to check on whether patients are at risk of taking two medicines with the same action (or which contain the same ingredient) at the same time. This is of special concern in the case of medicines that can also be bought over the counter (e.g. aspirin and paracetamol). Pharmacists reduce this risk to some extent by making sure that the words 'aspirin' or 'aspirin and paracetamol' appear on relevant preparations. A check on the patient's medicines (including cough and cold preparations) might prevent the patient inadvertently taking duplicate doses of aspirin or paracetamol.

Prices

Net prices have been included in the NPF to provide an indication of relative cost. These prices are **not** suitable for quoting to patients since they do not include the pharmacist's professional fee and other allowances, nor do they include VAT.

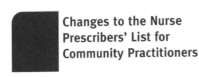

Changes to the Nurse Prescribers' List for Community Practitioners

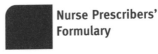

Nurse Prescribers' Formulary

Nurse Prescribers' Formulary for Community Practitioners

List of preparations approved by the Secretary of State which may be prescribed on form FP10P (form HS21(N) in Northern Ireland, form GP10(N) in Scotland, forms WP10CN and WP10PN in Wales) by Nurses for National Health Service patients.

Community Practitioners who have completed the necessary training may only prescribe items appearing in the nurse prescribers' list set out below. Community Practitioner Nurse Prescribers are recommended to prescribe generically, except where this would not be clinically appropriate or where there is no approved generic name.

Additions

Medicinal preparations added to Nurse Prescribers' List since 2011

Emollients as listed below:
Doublebase® Dayleve Gel
Macrogol Oral Liquid, Compound, NPF

Deletions

Preparations deleted from the Nurse Prescribers' List since 2011

Dimeticone Cream (*Vasogen*)

Folic Acid 400 micrograms/5 mL Oral Solution, NPF

Phosphate Suppositories, NPF

Zinc Cream, BP

Zinc Ointment, BP

Significant dose changes

Significant changes in dose statements introduced into NPF 2013–2015

Compound Macrogol Oral Powder, p. 9

Compound Macrogol Oral Powder, Half-Strength, p. 10

Medicinal Preparations

Almond Oil Ear Drops, BP
Arachis Oil Enema, NPF
[1]Aspirin Tablets, Dispersible, 300 mg, BP
Bisacodyl Suppositories, BP (includes 5-mg and 10-mg strengths)
Bisacodyl Tablets, BP
Catheter Maintenance Solution, Sodium Chloride, NPF
Catheter Maintenance Solution, 'Solution G', NPF
Catheter Maintenance Solution, 'Solution R', NPF
Chlorhexidine Gluconate Alcoholic Solutions containing at least 0.05%
Chlorhexidine Gluconate Aqueous Solutions containing at least 0.05%
Choline Salicylate Dental Gel, BP
Clotrimazole Cream 1%, BP
Co-danthramer Capsules, NPF
Co-danthramer Capsules, Strong, NPF
Co-danthramer Oral Suspension, NPF
Co-danthramer Oral Suspension, Strong, NPF
Co-danthrusate Capsules, BP
Co-danthrusate Oral Suspension, NPF
Crotamiton Cream, BP
Crotamiton Lotion, BP
Dimeticone barrier creams containing at least 10%
Dimeticone Lotion, NPF
Docusate Capsules, BP
Docusate Enema, NPF
Docusate Oral Solution, BP
Docusate Oral Solution, Paediatric, BP
Econazole Cream 1%, BP
Emollients as listed below:
Aquadrate® 10% w/w Cream
Arachis Oil, BP
Balneum® Plus Cream
Cetraben® Emollient Cream
Dermamist®
Diprobase® Cream
Diprobase® Ointment
Doublebase®
Doublebase® Dayleve Gel
E45® Cream
E45® Itch Relief Cream
Emulsifying Ointment, BP

---

1. Max. 96 tablets; max. pack size 32 tablets

Eucerin® Intensive 10% w/w Urea Treatment Cream
Eucerin® Intensive 10% w/w Urea Treatment Lotion
Hydromol® Cream
Hydromol® Intensive
[1]Hydromol® Ointment
Hydrous Ointment, BP
Lipobase®
Liquid and White Soft Paraffin Ointment, NPF
Neutrogena® Norwegian Formula Dermatological Cream
Nutraplus® Cream
Oilatum® Cream
Oilatum® Junior Cream
Paraffin, White Soft, BP
Paraffin, Yellow Soft, BP
Ultrabase®
Unguentum M®
Emollient Bath Additives and Shower Preparations as listed below:
   Aqueous Cream, BP
   [2]Balneum®
   [2]Balneum Plus® Bath Oil
   Cetraben® Emollient Bath Additive
   Dermalo® Bath Emollient
   Diprobath®
   Doublebase® Emollient Bath Additive
   Doublebase® Emollient Shower Gel
   Doublebase® Emollient Wash Gel
   Hydromol® Bath and Shower Emollient
   Oilatum® Emollient
   Oilatum® Junior Bath Additive
   Oilatum® Gel
   Zerolatum® Emollient Medicinal Bath Oil
Folic Acid Tablets 400 micrograms, BP
Glycerol Suppositories, BP
[3]Ibuprofen Oral Suspension, BP
[3]Ibuprofen Tablets, BP
Ispaghula Husk Granules, BP
Ispaghula Husk Granules, Effervescent, BP
Ispaghula Husk Oral Powder, BP
Lactulose Solution, BP
Lidocaine Ointment, BP
Lidocaine and Chlorhexidine Gel, BP
Macrogol Oral Liquid, Compound, NPF
Macrogol Oral Powder, Compound, NPF
Macrogol Oral Powder, Compound, Half-strength, NPF
Magnesium Hydroxide Mixture, BP
Magnesium Sulfate Paste, BP
Malathion aqueous lotions containing at least 0.5%
Mebendazole Oral Suspension, NPF
Mebendazole Tablets, NPF
Methylcellulose Tablets, BP
Miconazole Cream 2%, BP
Miconazole Oromucosal Gel, BP
Mouthwash Solution-tablets, NPF
Nicotine Inhalation Cartridge for Oromucosal Use, NPF
Nicotine Lozenge, NPF
Nicotine Medicated Chewing Gum, NPF
Nicotine Nasal Spray, NPF
Nicotine Oral Spray, NPF
Nicotine Sublingual Tablets, NPF

Nicotine Transdermal Patches, NPF
Nystatin Oral Suspension, BP
Olive Oil Ear Drops, BP
Paracetamol Oral Suspension, BP (includes 120 mg/5 mL and 250 mg/5 mL strengths—both of which are available as sugar-free formulations)
[4]Paracetamol Tablets, BP
[4]Paracetamol Tablets, Soluble, BP (includes 120-mg and 500-mg tablets)
Permethrin Cream, NPF
Phosphates Enema, BP
Piperazine and Senna Powder, NPF
Povidone–Iodine Solution, BP
Senna Oral Solution, NPF
Senna Tablets, BP
Senna and Ispaghula Granules, NPF
Sodium Chloride Solution, Sterile, BP
Sodium Citrate Compound Enema, NPF
Sodium Picosulfate Capsules, NPF
Sodium Picosulfate Elixir, NPF
Spermicidal contraceptives as listed below:
   Gygel® Contraceptive Jelly
Sterculia Granules, NPF
Sterculia and Frangula Granules, NPF
Titanium Ointment, BP
Water for Injections, BP
Zinc and Castor Oil Ointment, BP
Zinc Oxide and Dimeticone Spray, NPF
Zinc Oxide Impregnated Medicated Bandage, NPF
Zinc Oxide Impregnated Medicated Stocking, NPF
Zinc Paste Bandage, BP 1993
Zinc Paste and Ichthammol Bandage, BP 1993

Appliances and Reagents (including Wound Management Products)

Community Practitioner Nurse Prescribers in England, Wales and Northern Ireland can prescribe any appliance or reagent in the relevant Drug Tariff. In the Scottish Drug Tariff, Appliances and Reagents which may **not** be prescribed by Nurses are annotated **Nx**.

Appliances (including Contraceptive Devices[5]) as listed in Part IXA of the Drug Tariff (Part III of the Northern Ireland Drug Tariff, Part 3 (Appliances) and Part 2 (Dressings) of the Scottish Drug Tariff)

Incontinence Appliances as listed in Part IXB of the Drug Tariff (Part III of the Northern Ireland Drug Tariff, Part 5 of the Scottish Drug Tariff)

Stoma Appliances and Associated Products as listed in Part IXC of the Drug Tariff (Part III of the Northern Ireland Drug Tariff, Part 6 of the Scottish Drug Tariff)

---

1. Included in the Drug Tariff (Part IXA), the Scottish Drug Tariff (Part 2) and the Northern Ireland Drug Tariff (part III)
2. Except pack sizes that are not to be prescribed under the NHS (see Part XVIIIA of the Drug Tariff, Part XI of the Northern Ireland Drug Tariff)
3. Except for indications and doses that are PoM
4. Max. 96 tablets; max. pack size 32 tablets
5. Nurse Prescribers in Family Planning Clinics—where it is not appropriate for nurse prescribers in family planning clinics to prescribe contraceptive devices using form FP10P (forms WP10CN and WP10PN in Wales), they may prescribe using the same system as doctors in the clinic

Chemical Reagents as listed in Part IXR of the Drug Tariff (Part II of the Northern Ireland Drug Tariff, Part 9 of the Scottish Drug Tariff)

The Drug Tariffs can be accessed online at:

National Health Service Drug Tariff for England and Wales: www.ppa.org.uk/ppa/edt_intro.htm

Health and Personal Social Services for Northern Ireland Drug Tariff: www.dhsspsni.gov.uk/pas-tariff

Scottish Drug Tariff: www.isdscotland.org/Health-topics/Prescribing-and-Medicines/Scottish-Drug-Tariff

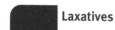

Laxatives

Corresponds to BNF section 1.6.

Before prescribing laxatives it is important to be sure that the patient *is* constipated and that the constipation is *not* secondary to an underlying undiagnosed complaint.

It is also important for those who complain of constipation to understand that bowel habit can vary considerably in frequency without doing harm. Some people tend to consider themselves constipated if they do not have a bowel movement each day. A useful definition of constipation is the passage of hard stools less frequently than the patient's own normal pattern and this can be explained to the patient.

Misconceptions about bowel habits have led to excessive laxative use. Abuse may lead to hypokalaemia. *Simple constipation* is usually relieved by increasing the intake of dietary fibre and fluids.

Laxatives should generally be **avoided** except where straining will exacerbate a condition (such as angina) or increase the risk of rectal bleeding as in haemorrhoids. Laxatives are also of value in *drug-induced constipation*, for the *expulsion of parasites* after anthelmintic treatment, and to clear the alimentary tract *before surgery and radiological procedures*. Prolonged treatment of constipation is sometimes necessary.

Children Laxatives should be prescribed by a healthcare professional experienced in the management of constipation in children. Delays of greater than 3 days between stools may increase the likelihood of pain on passing hard stools leading to anal fissure, anal spasm and eventually to a learned response to avoid defaecation. Increased fluid and fibre intake may be sufficient to regulate bowel action.

> Community Practitioner nurse prescribers should discuss with the doctor before prescribing a laxative for a child

Laxatives can be divided into four main groups: *bulk-forming laxatives, stimulant laxatives, faecal softeners*, and *osmotic laxatives*. This simple classification, however, disguises the fact that some laxatives have complex actions.

Bulk-forming laxatives

Bulk-forming laxatives relieve constipation by increasing faecal mass which stimulates peristalsis. Patients should be advised that the full effect may take some days to develop. In nursing practice they are particularly useful in the management of patients with *colostomy, ileostomy, haemorrhoids*, and *anal fissure*. Methylcellulose tablets are licensed for other indications including diarrhoea and obesity but nurse prescribers should prescribe them **only** for constipation.

▮ BULK-FORMING LAXATIVES

Indications constipation, see also notes above

Cautions adequate fluid intake should be maintained to avoid intestinal obstruction—it may be necessary to supervise elderly or debilitated patients or those with intestinal narrowing or decreased motility

Contra-indications difficulty in swallowing, intestinal obstruction, colonic atony, faecal impaction; avoid methylcellulose in infective bowel disease

Pregnancy manufacturer of *Normacol Plus®* advises avoid

Breast-feeding manufacturer of *Normacol Plus®* advises avoid

Side-effects flatulence, abdominal distension; gastro-intestinal obstruction or impaction; hypersensitivity reported

Dose
● See preparations, below

> **Counselling**
> Preparations that swell in contact with liquid should always be carefully swallowed with water and should not be taken immediately before going to bed

◀*Prescribe as:*

Ispaghula Husk Granules (Isogel)

Granules, brown, sugar- and gluten-free, ispaghula husk 90%, net price 200 g = £3.24.

Dose 2 level 5-mL spoonfuls in water once or twice daily, preferably at mealtimes; CHILD (but see notes above) 6–12 years 1 level 5-mL spoonful in water once or twice daily, preferably at mealtimes

Note May be difficult to obtain

Ispaghula Husk Oral Powder (Regulan)

Powder, beige, sugar- and gluten-free, ispaghula husk 3.4 g/5.85-g sachet (orange or lemon/lime flavour), net price 30 sachets = £2.44.

Excipients include aspartame (see BNF section 9.4.1)

Dose 1 sachet in 150 mL water 1–3 times daily, preferably after meals; CHILD (but see notes above) 6–12 years ½–1 level 5-mL spoonful in water 1–3 times daily, preferably after meals

Effervescent Ispaghula Husk Granules (Fybogel)

Granules, buff, effervescent, sugar- and gluten-free, ispaghula husk 3.5 g/sachet, net price 30 sachets (lemon or orange flavour or plain) = £1.84

Excipients include aspartame 16 mg/sachet (see BNF section 9.4.1)

Dose 1 sachet or 2 level 5-mL spoonfuls in water twice daily, preferably after meals; CHILD (but see notes above) 6–12 years ½–1 level 5-mL spoonful in water twice daily, preferably after meals

Effervescent Ispaghula Husk Granules (Ispagel Orange)

Granules, beige, effervescent, sugar- and gluten-free, ispaghula husk 3.5 g/sachet (orange flavour), net price 30 sachets = £1.69.

Excipients include aspartame (see BNF section 9.4.1)

Dose 1 sachet in water 1–3 times daily, preferably after meals; CHILD (but see notes above) 6–12 years half adult dose

Methylcellulose Tablets

Tablets, pink, scored, methylcellulose '450' 500 mg, net price 112-tab pack = £3.22. *Proprietary product: Celevac tablets*

Dose 3–6 tablets twice daily with at least 300 mL of liquid

Sterculia Granules

Granules, coated, gluten-free, sterculia 62%, net price 500 g = £6.85; 60 × 7-g sachets = £5.77. *Proprietary product: Normacol*

Dose 1–2 heaped 5-mL spoonfuls or contents of 1–2 sachets, washed down without chewing with plenty of liquid once or twice daily after meals; CHILD (but see notes above) 6–12 years half adult dose

Sterculia and Frangula Granules

Granules, brown, coated, gluten-free, sterculia 62%, frangula (standardised) 8%, net price 500 g = £7.32; 60 × 7-g sachets = £6.16. *Proprietary product: Normacol Plus*

Dose 1–2 heaped 5-mL spoonfuls *or* contents of 1–2 sachets, washed down without chewing with plenty of liquid once or twice daily after meals

Stimulant laxatives

Stimulant laxatives increase intestinal motility and are used in functional constipation that has not responded to dietary measures.

Stimulant laxatives often cause abdominal cramp. They should be avoided in intestinal obstruction, and excessive use can cause diarrhoea and related effects such as hypokalaemia.

> Community Practitioner nurse prescribers should discuss with the doctor before prescribing a laxative for a child

> Cross-references to the BNF are provided but nurse prescribers may only prescribe those items that are listed on the Nurse Prescribers' list.

■ BISACODYL

Indications constipation; tablets act in 10–12 hours; suppositories act in 20–60 minutes

Cautions see notes on stimulant laxatives

Contra-indications see notes on stimulant laxatives; acute surgical abdominal conditions, acute inflammatory bowel disease, severe dehydration

Side-effects see notes on stimulant laxatives; nausea and vomiting; colitis also reported; *suppositories*, local irritation

Dose
● See under preparations, below

◢*Prescribe as:*

Bisacodyl Tablets 5 mg

Tablets, enteric coated, bisacodyl 5 mg. Net price 100 = £3.43

Dose 1–2 tablets at night, increased if necessary to max. 20 mg at night; CHILD (but see notes above) 4–10 years (on doctor's advice only) 1 tablet at night, over 10 years 1–2 tablets at night

Bisacodyl Suppositories 10 mg

Suppositories, bisacodyl 10 mg. Net price 12 = £3.30

Dose 1 suppository rectally in the morning; CHILD over 10 years (but see notes above) 1 suppository rectally in the morning

Bisacodyl Paediatric Suppositories 5 mg

Paediatric suppositories, bisacodyl 5 mg. Net price 5 = 99p

Dose CHILD (but see notes above) 4–10 years 1 suppository rectally in the morning (on doctor's advice only)

■ DANTRON

(Danthron)

Indications in consultation with doctor, only for: constipation in terminally ill patients of all ages; acts within 6–12 hours

Cautions see notes on stimulant laxatives; avoid prolonged contact with skin (as in incontinent patients)—

risk of irritation and excoriation; *rodent* studies indicate potential carcinogenic risk

Contra-indications see notes on stimulant laxatives

Pregnancy manufacturers of co-danthramer and co-danthrusate advise avoid—no information available

Breast-feeding manufacturers of co-danthramer and co-danthrusate advise avoid—limited information available

Side-effects see notes on stimulant laxatives; urine may be coloured red

Dose
● See under preparations

◢*Prescribe as:*

Co-danthramer Capsules [PoM]

Capsules, co-danthramer 25/200 (dantron 25 mg, poloxamer '188' 200 mg). Net price 60-cap pack = £12.86

Dose (restricted indications, see above) 1–2 capsules at bedtime; CHILD 1 capsule at bedtime

Strong Co-danthramer Capsules [PoM]

Capsules, co-danthramer 37.5/500 (dantron 37.5 mg, poloxamer '188' 500 mg). Net price 60-cap pack = £15.55

Dose (restricted indications, see above) 1–2 capsules at bedtime; CHILD under 12 years not recommended

Co-danthramer Oral Suspension [PoM]

Oral suspension, co-danthramer 25/200 in 5 mL (dantron 25 mg, poloxamer '188' 200 mg/5 mL). Net price 300 mL = £11.27, 1 litre = £37.57

Dose (restricted indications, see above) 5–10 mL at night; CHILD 2.5–5 mL

Strong Co-danthramer Oral Suspension [PoM]

Strong oral suspension, co-danthramer 75/1000 in 5 mL (dantron 75 mg, poloxamer '188' 1 g/5 mL). Net price 300 mL = £30.13

Dose (restricted indications, see above) 5 mL at night; CHILD under 12 years not recommended

Co-danthrusate Capsules [PoM]

Capsules, co-danthrusate 50/60 (dantron 50 mg, docusate sodium 60 mg). Net price 63-cap pack = £20.24

Dose (restricted indications, see above) 1–3 capsules, usually at night; CHILD 6–12 years 1 capsule at night

Co-danthrusate Oral Suspension [PoM]

Oral suspension, yellow, co-danthrusate 50/60 in 5 mL (dantron 50 mg, docusate sodium 60 mg/5 mL). Net price 200 mL = £17.95.

Dose (restricted indications, see above) 5–15 mL at night; CHILD 6–12 years 5 mL at night

■ DOCUSATE SODIUM

(Dioctyl Sodium Sulphosuccinate)

Indications constipation (oral preparations act within 1–2 days)

Cautions see notes on stimulant laxatives; do not give with liquid paraffin; rectal preparations not indicated if haemorrhoids or anal fissure

Contra-indications see notes on stimulant laxatives

Pregnancy not known to be harmful—manufacturer advises caution

Breast-feeding present in milk following oral administration—manufacturer advises caution; rectal administration not known to be harmful

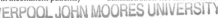

Side-effects see notes on stimulant laxatives; also rash

Dose

- See under preparations

    Note Docusate preparations probably also have faecal softening effect.

◢*Prescribe as:*

Docusate Capsules 100 mg

Capsules, yellow/white, docusate sodium 100 mg, net price 30-cap pack = £2.09, 100-cap pack = £6.98. *Proprietary product: Dioctyl Capsules*

Dose up to 5 capsules daily in divided doses

Docusate Oral Solution 50 mg/5 mL

Oral solution, sugar-free, docusate sodium 50 mg/5 mL. Net price 300-mL = £5.49. *Proprietary product: Docusol Adult Solution*

Dose up to 50 mL daily in divided doses

Paediatric Docusate Oral Solution 12.5 mg/5 mL

Paediatric oral solution, sugar-free, docusate sodium 12.5 mg/5 mL. Net price 300 mL = £5.29. *Proprietary product: Docusol Paediatric Solution*

Dose CHILD (but see notes above) 6 months–2 years 5 mL 3 times daily, adjusted according to response, 2–12 years 5–10 mL 3 times daily, adjusted according to response

Docusate Enema

Enema, docusate sodium 120 mg in 10-g single-dose disposable packs. Net price 10-g unit = 66p. *Proprietary product: Norgalax Micro-enema*

Dose ADULT and CHILD (but see notes above) over 12 years, 10-g unit

◢ GLYCEROL

(Glycerin)

Indications constipation

Dose

- See under preparations

◢*Prescribe as:*

Glycerol Suppositories

(Synonym: Glycerin Suppositories)

Suppositories, gelatin 140 mg, glycerol (glycerin) 700 mg/g. Net price 12 × 1-g = 89p; 12 × 2-g = 89p; 12 × 4-g = £3.16

Dose 1 suppository moistened with water before use, when required

The usual sizes are INFANT under 1 year, small (1-g mould), CHILD 1–12 years medium (2-g mould), ADULT and CHILD over 12 years, large (4-g mould)

◢ SENNA

Indications constipation (acts within 8–12 hours)

Cautions see notes on stimulant laxatives

Contra-indications see notes on stimulant laxatives

Breast-feeding not known to be harmful

Side-effects see notes on stimulant laxatives

Dose

- See under preparations

◢*Prescribe as:*

Senna Tablets

Tablets, total sennosides (calculated as sennoside B) 7.5 mg. Net price 60 = £4.18

Dose 2–4 tablets, usually at bedtime; initial dose should be low and then gradually increased; CHILD (but see notes above) 6–12 years, half adult dose in the morning

Note For senna tablets on general sale to the public lower dose recommended

Senna Oral Solution

Syrup, brown, total sennosides (calculated as sennoside B) 7.5 mg/5 mL. Net price 500 mL = £2.69 *Proprietary product: Senokot Syrup*

Dose 10–20 mL, usually at bedtime; CHILD (but see notes above) 2–6 years 2.5–5 mL once daily, 6–12 years, 5–10 mL once daily

Note For senna oral solution on general sale to the public lower dose recommended

Senna and Ispaghula Granules

Granules, coated, senna fruit 12.4%, ispaghula 54.2%. Contain ispaghula as a bulk laxative. Net price 400 g = £8.99. *Proprietary product: Manevac Granules*

Dose ADULT and CHILD (but see notes above) over 12 years, 1–2 level 5-mL spoonfuls at night with at least 150 mL water, fruit juice, milk or warm drink

Counselling Preparations that swell in contact with liquid should always be carefully swallowed with water and should not be taken immediately before going to bed

◢ SODIUM PICOSULFATE

(Sodium Picosulphate)

Indications constipation (acts within 6–12 hours)

Cautions see notes on stimulant laxatives; active inflammatory bowel disease (avoid if fulminant)

Contra-indications see notes on stimulant laxatives; severe dehydration

Breast-feeding not known to be present in milk but manufacturer advises avoid unless potential benefit outweighs risk

Side-effects see notes on stimulant laxatives; also nausea and vomiting

Dose

- See under preparations

◢*Prescribe as:*

Sodium Picosulfate Capsules

Capsules, sodium picosulfate 2.5 mg, net price 20-cap pack = £2.03, 50-cap pack = £2.87. *Proprietary product: [1]Dulcolax Pico Perles*

Dose 2–4 capsules at night; CHILD (but see notes above) 4–10 years 1–2 capsules at night (on doctor's advice only), adjusted according to response, over 10 years 2–4 capsules at night, adjusted according to response

1. The brand name *Dulcolax®* is also used for bisacodyl tablets and suppositories

Sodium Picosulfate Elixir

Elixir, sodium picosulfate 5 mg/5 mL. Net price 100 mL = £1.89. *Proprietary product: [2]Dulcolax Pico Liquid*

Dose 5–10 mL at night; CHILD (but see notes above), under 4 years 250 micrograms/kg (max. 5 mg) at night (on doctor's advice only), 4–10 years 2.5–5 mL at night (on doctor's advice only), over 10 years 5–10 mL at night, adjusted according to response

2. The brand name *Dulcolax®* is also used for bisacodyl tablets and suppositories

Faecal softeners

Faecal softeners, such as enemas containing arachis oil (ground-nut oil, peanut oil), lubricate and soften impacted faeces and promote a bowel movement.

◢ ARACHIS OIL

Indications constipation, see also notes above

Dose

- See under preparation

Prescribe as:

Arachis Oil Enema

Enema, arachis (peanut) oil in 130-mL single-dose
disposable packs. Net price 130 mL = £7.98

Dose to soften impacted faeces, 130 mL; the enema should be
warmed before use; CHILD on doctor's advice only

Osmotic laxatives

Osmotic laxatives increase the amount of water in the
large bowel, either by drawing fluid from the body into
the bowel or by retaining the fluid they were administered with.

Lactulose is a semi-synthetic disaccharide which is not
absorbed from the gastro-intestinal tract. It is contra-
indicated in galactosaemia and in intestinal obstruction.

Macrogol (polyethylene glycol) may be used by mouth
for constipation and the short-term treatment of faecal
impaction. It is important that the initial assessment of
faecal impaction is undertaken by a doctor. A multi-
disciplinary approach may be needed after disimpaction
for investigation or for maintenance laxative therapy.
Macrogols sequester fluid in the bowel; giving fluid with
macrogols may reduce the dehydrating effect sometimes seen with osmotic laxatives.

Magnesium hydroxide mixture is suitable for occasional use provided an adequate fluid intake is maintained after it has been given. It may be used when a
rapid action is required but should be prescribed with
caution because it is often abused.

Phosphate enemas are useful in bowel clearance
before radiology, endoscopy, and surgery.

> Community Practitioner nurse prescribers should
> discuss with the doctor before prescribing a laxative
> for a child

◢ LACTULOSE

Indications constipation (may take up to 48 hours to
act)

Cautions lactose intolerance; **interactions:** BNF
Appendix 1 (lactulose)

Contra-indications galactosaemia, intestinal obstruction

Pregnancy not known to be harmful

Side-effects nausea (can be reduced by administration with water, fruit juice or with meals), vomiting,
flatulence, cramps, and abdominal discomfort

Dose
● See under preparation

Prescribe as:

Lactulose Solution

Solution, lactulose 3.1–3.7 g/5 mL with other
ketoses. Net price 300-mL pack = £2.04, 500-mL
pack = £3.23, 10 × 15 mL sachet pack = £2.50

Dose initially 15 mL twice daily, adjusted according to response;
CHILD (but see notes above) under 1 year 2.5 mL twice daily, 1–5
years 5 mL twice daily, 5–10 years 10 mL twice daily

◢ MACROGOLS
(Polyethylene glycols)

Indications constipation; faecal impaction (**only after**
initial assessment by medical practitioner)

Cautions discontinue if symptoms of fluid and
electrolyte disturbance; see also preparations below

Contra-indications intestinal perforation or obstruction, paralytic ileus, severe inflammatory conditions
of the intestinal tract (such as Crohn's disease,
ulcerative colitis, and toxic megacolon)

Pregnancy manufacturers advice use only if essential—no information available

Breast-feeding manufacturers advice use only if
essential—no information available

Side-effects abdominal distension and pain, nausea,
flatulence

Dose
● See under preparations

Prescribe as:

Compound Macrogol Oral Liquid

Oral concentrate, macrogol '3350' (polyethylene glycol '3350') 13.125 g, sodium bicarbonate 178.5 mg,
sodium chloride 350.7 mg, potassium chloride
46.6 mg/25 mL, net price 500 mL (orange flavoured)
= £4.45. *Proprietary product: Movicol Liquid*

Note 25 mL of oral concentrate when diluted with 100 mL
water provides K$^+$ 5.4 mmol/litreDose chronic constipation,
ADULT and CHILD (but see notes above) over 12 years, 25 mL 1–3
times daily usually for up to 2 weeks; maintenance, 25 mL 1–2
times daily

Counselling 25 mL of oral concentrate to be diluted with
half a glass (approx. 100 mL) of water. After dilution the
solution should be discarded if unused after 24 hours

Compound Macrogol Oral Powder

Oral powder, macrogol '3350' (polyethylene glycol
'3350') 13.125 g, sodium bicarbonate 178.5 mg, sodium chloride 350.7 mg, potassium chloride 46.6 mg/
sachet, net price 20-sachet pack (lime- and lemon-,
or orange-, or plain-flavoured) = £4.45, 30-sachet
pack (lime- and lemon-, or orange-, or chocolate-,
or plain-flavoured) = £6.68, 50-sachet pack (lime-
and lemon-, or plain-flavoured) = £11.13. *Proprietary
products: Laxido Orange, Molaxole, Movicol*

Note Amount of potassium chloride varies according to
flavour of *Movicol®* as follows: plain-flavour (sugar-free) =
50.2 mg/sachet; lime and lemon flavour = 46.6 mg/sachet;
chocolate flavour = 31.7 mg/sachet. 1 sachet when
reconstituted with 125 mL water provides K$^+$ 5.4 mmol/litre

Not to be confused with preparations also containing sodium
sulfate which are used for bowel cleansing before surgery
and bowel procedures

Cautions patients with cardiovascular impairment should not
take more than 2 sachets in any 1 hour

Dose chronic constipation, ADULT and CHILD (but see notes
above) over 12 years, 1–3 sachets daily in divided doses usually
for up to 2 weeks; maintenance, 1–2 sachets daily

Faecal impaction (**important**: initial assessment by doctor),
ADULT and CHILD (but see notes above) over 12 years, 4
sachets on first day, then increased in steps of 2 sachets daily
to max. 8 sachets daily; total daily dose to be drunk within a 6
hour period; usual max. 3 days; after disimpaction, consider
whether to refer to a doctor for investigation or maintenance
laxative therapy

Counselling Contents of each sachet to be dissolved in half
a glass (approx. 125 mL) of water; after reconstitution the
solution should be kept in a refrigerator and discarded if
unused after 6 hours

Compound Macrogol Oral Powder, Half-Strength

Oral powder, macrogol '3350' (polyethylene glycol '3350') 6.563 g, sodium bicarbonate 89.3 mg, sodium chloride 175.4 mg, potassium chloride 23.3 mg/sachet, net price 20-sachet pack (lime and lemon flavour) = £2.92, 30-sachet pack = £4.38. *Proprietary product: Movicol-Half*

Note *Movicol Paediatric Plain* is PoM and is **not** on the NPF list

Cautions patients with cardiovascular impairment should not take more than 4 sachets in any 1 hour

Dose chronic constipation, ADULT and CHILD (but see notes above) over 12 years 2–6 sachets daily in divided doses usually for up to 2 weeks; maintenance, 2–4 sachets daily

Faecal impaction (**important**: initial assessment by doctor), ADULT and CHILD (but see notes above) over 12 years 8 sachets on first day, then increased in steps of 4 sachets daily to max. 16 sachets daily; total daily dose to be drunk within a 6 hour period; usual max. 3 days; after disimpaction, consider whether to refer to a doctor for investigation or maintenance laxative therapy

Counselling Contents of each sachet to be dissolved in quarter of a glass (approx. 60–65 mL) of water; after reconstitution the solution should be kept in a refrigerator and discarded if unused after 6 hours

MAGNESIUM HYDROXIDE

Indications constipation

Cautions elderly and debilitated; see also notes above; interactions: see BNF Appendix 1 (antacids)

Contra-indications acute gastro-intestinal conditions

Hepatic impairment avoid in hepatic coma if risk of renal failure

Renal impairment avoid or reduce dose; increased risk of toxicity

Side-effects colic

Dose
- See under preparation

◀*Prescribe as:*

Magnesium Hydroxide Mixture

(Synonym: Cream of Magnesia)

Mixture, aqueous suspension containing about 8% of hydrated magnesium oxide. Do not store in a cold place

Dose constipation, ADULT and CHILD over 12 years, 30–45 mL with water at bedtime when required; CHILD (but see notes above) 3–12 years, 5–10 mL with water at bedtime when required

PHOSPHATES (RECTAL)

Indications rectal use in constipation, see also notes above

Cautions elderly and debilitated; electrolyte disturbances, congestive heart failure, ascites, uncontrolled hypertension, maintain adequate hydration

Contra-indications acute gastro-intestinal conditions (including gastro-intestinal obstruction, inflammatory bowel disease, and conditions associated with increased colonic absorption)

Renal impairment use with caution

Side-effects local irritation; electrolyte disturbances

Dose
- See under preparations

◀*Prescribe as:*

Phosphates Enema (Formula B)

Enema, sodium dihydrogen phosphate dihydrate 12.8 g, disodium phosphate dodecahydrate 10.24 g/128 mL. Net price 128 mL with standard tube = £2.98, with long rectal tube = £3.98

Dose 128 mL; CHILD (but see notes above) over 3 years, reduced according to body weight (under 3 years not recommended)

Phosphates Enema (Fleet)

Enema, sodium acid phosphate 21.4 g, sodium phosphate 9.4 g/118 mL. Net price single-dose pack (standard tube) = 68p

Dose ADULT and CHILD over 12 years, 118 mL; CHILD (but see notes above) 3–12 years, on doctor's advice only (under 3 years not recommended)

SODIUM CITRATE (RECTAL)

Indications rectal use in constipation

Cautions elderly and debilitated

Contra-indications acute gastro-intestinal conditions

Dose
- See under preparations

◀*Prescribe as:*

Sodium Citrate Compound Enema

Enema, sodium citrate 450 mg with other ingredients including glycerol, sorbitol and an anionic surfactant in a 5-mL single-dose disposable pack. *Proprietary products: Micolette Micro-enema* (net price 5-mL pack = 41p), *Micralax Micro-enema* (5-mL pack = 41p), *Relaxit Micro-enema* (5-mL pack = 43p)

Dose ADULT and CHILD (but see notes above) over 3 years, 5 mL (under 3 years not recommended)

Gloves

GLOVES

EMA Film Gloves, Disposable

Gloves, small, medium, or large. Net price pack of 30 = £2.43, pack of 100 = £3.31. *Proprietary product: Dispos-A-Gloves*

For use as a barrier during manual evacuation of the bowel

Nitrile Gloves

Gloves, small, medium, large, or extra large, net price pack of 50 = £3.89

Polythene Gloves

Gloves, net price pack of 25 = 59p.

For use as occlusives with medicated creams

Analgesics

Corresponds to BNF section 4.7.1 (non-opioid analgesics) and 10.1.1 (non-steroidal anti-inflammatory drugs)

The **non-opioid** analgesics **aspirin**, **ibuprofen** and **paracetamol** are particularly suitable for pain in musculoskeletal conditions, whereas the opioid analgesics are more suitable for moderate to severe visceral pain. Aspirin, ibuprofen, and paracetamol are effective analgesics for the relief of *mild to moderate pain*. Their familiar role as household remedies should not detract from their considerable value as analgesics; they are also of value in some forms of *severe chronic pain*.

Combinations of aspirin or paracetamol with an opioid analgesic (such as codeine) are commonly used but their advantages have not been substantiated (and they are not on the Nurse Prescribers' List). Any additional pain relief that they might provide can be at the cost of *increased side-effects caused by the opioid component* (constipation, in particular).

> When prescribing aspirin or paracetamol it is important to make sure that the patient is not already taking an aspirin- or a paracetamol-containing preparation (possibly bought over-the-counter).

Aspirin

Aspirin is indicated for mild to moderate pain including headache, transient musculoskeletal pain, and dysmenorrhoea; it has anti-inflammatory properties which may be useful, and is an antipyretic. The main side-effect is gastric irritation; rarely, gastric bleeding can be a serious complication. Aspirin increases bleeding time and must **not** be prescribed as an analgesic to patients receiving anticoagulants such as warfarin. Aspirin is also associated with bronchospasm and allergic reactions, particularly in patients with asthma. It should **not** be prescribed for patients with a history of hypersensitivity to aspirin or any other non-steroidal anti-inflammatory drug (NSAID)—which includes those in whom asthma, angioedema, urticaria or rhinitis have been precipitated by aspirin or another NSAID. Aspirin should **not** be prescribed for children and adolescents **under the age of 16 years** owing to its association with Reye's syndrome.

> Other uses
>
> Since aspirin decreases platelet aggregation, it is prescribed in low doses (e.g. 75–150 mg daily) to prevent cerebrovascular or cardiovascular disease. Aspirin is also *occasionally* prescribed for rheumatic conditions. Community Practitioner nurse prescribers should **not** prescribe aspirin for these conditions.

ASPIRIN

Indications mild to moderate pain, pyrexia

Cautions asthma, allergic disease, dehydration; preferably avoid during fever or viral infection in adolescents (risk of Reye's syndrome, see below); elderly; G6PD-deficiency (acceptable in a dose of up to 1 g daily in most G6PD-deficient individuals); concomitant use of drugs that increase risk of bleeding; anaemia; thyrotoxicosis; **interactions**: see BNF Appendix 1 (aspirin)

Contra-indications children under 16 years (Reye's syndrome—see below); previous or active peptic ulceration, haemophilia; severe cardiac failure; not for treatment of gout

Hypersensitivity. Aspirin and other NSAIDs are **contra-indicated** in patients with a history of hypersensitivity to aspirin or any other NSAID—*which includes those* in whom attacks of *asthma, angioedema, urticaria or rhinitis* have been precipitated by aspirin or any other NSAID

Reye's Syndrome. Owing to an association with Reye's syndrome, aspirin-containing preparations should not be given to children under 16 years, unless specifically indicated, e.g. for Kawasaki syndrome.

Hepatic impairment avoid in severe impairment—increased risk of gastro-intestinal bleeding

Renal impairment use with caution; avoid in severe impairment; sodium and water retention; deterioration in renal function; increased risk of gastro-intestinal bleeding

Pregnancy high doses may be related to intrauterine growth restriction and teratogenic effects; impaired platelet function with risk of haemorrhage, and delayed onset and increased duration of labour with increased blood loss, can occur if used during delivery; avoid analgesic doses if possible in last few weeks (low doses probably not harmful); with high doses, closure of fetal ductus arteriosis in utero and possibly persistent pulmonary hypertension of newborn; kernicterus in jaundiced neonates

Breast-feeding avoid—possible risk of Reye's syndrome; regular use of high doses could impair platelet function and produce hypothrombinaemia in infant if neonatal vitamin K stores low

Side-effects generally mild and infrequent but high incidence of gastro-intestinal irritation with slight asymptomatic blood loss, blood disorders have occurred (including increased bleeding time), confusion, tinnitus, bronchospasm and skin reactions in hypersensitive patients; **overdosage**, immediate transfer to hospital essential

Dose

- Usual, 300–600 mg every 4–6 hours when necessary, not more than 2.4 g daily without doctor's advice; CHILD under 16 years not recommended (see Reye's syndrome above)

Prescribe as:

[1]**Dispersible Aspirin Tablets 300 mg** PoM

Dispersible tablets, aspirin 300 mg. Net price 32–tab pack = £1.29

Cautionary label added by pharmacist: dissolve or mix with water before taking and take with or after food

1. Nurse prescribers should prescribe packs containing no more than **32 tablets**, a max. of **3** packs of 32 tablets may be prescribed on each occasion: PoM but may be sold to the public under certain circumstances—for details see *Medicines, Ethics and Practice*, London, Pharmaceutical Press (always consult latest edition)

Ibuprofen

In single doses **ibuprofen** has analgesic activity comparable to that of paracetamol, but paracetamol is preferred for the management of pain, particularly in the elderly. Ibuprofen also has antipyretic properties. In regular dosage ibuprofen has a lasting analgesic and anti-inflammatory effect which makes it particularly useful for the treatment of pain associated with inflammation.

Like aspirin, ibuprofen has been associated with bronchospasm and allergic disorders; it is contra-indicated in patients with a history of hypersensitivity to aspirin or any other NSAID—which includes those in whom attacks of asthma, angioedema, urticaria or rhinitis have been precipitated by aspirin or any other NSAID.

The side-effects of ibuprofen include gastro-intestinal discomfort, nausea, diarrhoea, and occasionally bleeding and ulceration occur.

> **Other uses**
>
> Ibuprofen is prescribed for chronic inflammatory diseases. However, Community Practitioner nurse prescribers should not prescribe ibuprofen for indications or at doses other than those listed below.

IBUPROFEN

Indications rheumatic and muscular pain, headache, dental pain, fever (fever with discomfort in children), symptoms of colds and influenza; in adults also backache, neuralgia, migraine, dysmenorrhoea

Cautions allergic disorders (see Hypersensitivity below); coagulation defects; cardiac impairment, connective-tissue disorders, elderly (risk of serious side-effects); **interactions**: see BNF Appendix 1 (NSAIDs)

Contra-indications previous or active peptic ulceration, severe heart failure

Hypersensitivity **Contra-indicated** in patients with a history of hypersensitivity to aspirin or any other NSAID—*which includes those* in whom attacks of *asthma, angioedema, urticaria, or rhinitis* have been precipitated by aspirin or any other NSAID

Hepatic impairment use with caution—increased risk of gastro-intestinal bleeding and fluid retention; avoid in severe liver disease

Renal impairment use with caution—risk of deterioration of renal function; avoid in severe impairment

Pregnancy avoid unless potential benefit outweighs risk; avoid during third trimester because use is associated with a risk of closure of fetal ductus arteriosus *in utero* and possibly persistent pulmonary hypertension of the newborn; onset of labour may be delayed and its duration may be increased

Breast-feeding amount too small to be harmful but some manufacturers advise avoid

Side-effects gastro-intestinal discomfort including pain, indigestion and nausea; gastro-intestinal bleeding, bruising, bronchospasm, rashes, oedema, raised blood pressure, renal impairment; blood disorders reported; see BNF section 10.1.1 for other side-effects

Dose

- Initially 400 mg, then 200–400 mg every 4 hours, max. 1.2 g daily; if symptoms worsen or persist for more than 10 days refer to doctor

- Fever and pain in children, CHILD over 3 months and over 5 kg body-weight, 20–30 mg/kg daily in divided doses *or* 3–6 months 50 mg 3 times daily for max. 24 hours; 6–12 months 50 mg 3–4 times daily; 1–3 years 100 mg 3 times daily; 4–6 years 150 mg 3 times daily; 7–9 years 200 mg 3 times daily; 10–12 years 300 mg 3 times daily; refer to doctor if symptoms persist for more than 24 hours in child under 6 months or more than 3 days in child over 6 months

- Post-immunisation pyrexia, CHILD over 3 months 50 mg followed if necessary by second dose of 50 mg after 6 hours; if pyrexia persists refer to doctor

◢*Prescribe as:*

¹Ibuprofen [PoM]

Tablets, coated, ibuprofen 200 mg, net price 16 = 32p

Oral suspension, ibuprofen 100 mg/5 mL, net price 100 mL = £1.51

Note Sugar-free versions are available and can be ordered by specifying 'sugar-free' on the prescription

Cautionary label added by pharmacist: take with or after food

1. May be sold to the public under certain circumstances. Community Practitioner nurse prescribers should not prescribe outside the indications and doses above, other indications and doses are [PoM]

Paracetamol

Paracetamol is similar in efficacy to aspirin, but has no demonstrable anti-inflammatory activity. It is less irritant to the stomach and for that reason paracetamol is now generally preferred to aspirin, particularly in the elderly. It must be remembered, however, that overdosage with paracetamol (alone or as an ingredient of a combination product) is particularly dangerous.

PARACETAMOL

Indications mild to moderate pain, fever (fever with discomfort in children)

Cautions alcohol dependence; before administering, check when paracetamol last administered and cumulative paracetamol dose over previous 24 hours; **interactions**: see BNF Appendix 1 (paracetamol)

Hepatic impairment dose-related toxicity—avoid large doses

Renal impairment effervescent tables may be unsuitable due to sodium content

Pregnancy not known to be harmful

Breast-feeding amount too small to be harmful

Side-effects side-effects rare, but rashes and blood disorders (including thrombocytopenia, leucopenia, neutropenia) reported; **important**: liver damage (and less frequently renal damage) following **overdosage**, immediate transfer to hospital essential

Dose

- 0.5–1 g every 4–6 hours; max. 4 g daily

- CHILD 3–6 months 60 mg, 6 months–2 years 120 mg, 2–4 years 180 mg, 4–6 years 240 mg, 6–8 years 240–250 mg, 8–10 years 360–375 mg, 10–12 years 480–500 mg, 12–16 years 480–750 mg; these doses may be repeated every 4–6 hours when necessary; max. 4 doses in 24 hours

- Post-immunisation pyrexia, CHILD 2–3 months, 60 mg followed, if necessary, by second dose after 4–6 hours; if pyrexia persists refer to doctor

◢*Prescribe as:*

¹Paracetamol Tablets 500 mg [PoM]

Tablets, paracetamol 500 mg, net price 16 = 14p, 32 = 92p

Cautionary label added by pharmacist: Do not take more than 2 tablets at any one time. Do not take more than 8 in 24 hours. Do not take with any other paracetamol products. Talk to a doctor at once if you take too much of this medicine, even if you feel well

¹Soluble Paracetamol Tablets 500 mg [PoM]

Soluble tablets (Dispersible tablets), paracetamol 500 mg, net price 24 = £2.58

Cautionary label added by pharmacist: Do not take more than 2 tablets at any one time, do not take more than 8 in 24 hours, dissolve in water. Do not take with any other paracetamol products. Talk to a doctor at once if you take too much of this medicine, even if you feel well

Soluble Paracetamol Tablets 120 mg

Tablets (= Paediatric dispersible tablets), paracetamol 120 mg, net price 16-tab pack = 97p

Cautionary label added by pharmacist: Dissolve or mix with water before taking. Do not take with any other paracetamol products. Talk to a doctor at once if you take too much of this medicine, even if you feel well

Paracetamol Oral Suspension 120 mg/5 mL

Oral suspension (= Paediatric mixture), paracetamol 120 mg/5 mL, net price 100 mL = 72p

Note Sugar-free version can be ordered by specifying 'sugar-free' on the prescription

Cautionary label added by pharmacist: Do not take with any other paracetamol products. Talk to a doctor at once if you take too much of this medicine, even if you feel well. If a 60-mg dose is required the pharmacist will supply an oral syringe and advise on how to give a 2.5-mL dose

Paracetamol Oral Suspension 250 mg/5 mL

Oral suspension, (= Mixture) paracetamol 250 mg/5 mL, net price 100 mL = £1.30

Note Sugar-free version can be ordered by specifying 'sugar-free' on the prescription

Cautionary label added by pharmacist: Do not take with any other paracetamol products. Talk to a doctor at once if you take too much of this medicine, even if you feel well

 # Local anaesthetics

Corresponds to BNF section 15.2.

Lidocaine

Lidocaine (lignocaine) is effectively absorbed from mucous membranes and is a useful surface anaesthetic in concentrations of up to 10%. Except for surface anaesthesia, solutions should not usually exceed 1% in strength.

 ## LIDOCAINE HYDROCHLORIDE
(Lignocaine Hydrochloride)

Indications surface anaesthesia (**important**: consult with doctor), see notes above

Cautions absorbed through mucosa therefore special care if history of epilepsy, cardiac disease, respiratory disease, hepatic or renal impairment, myasthenia gravis, or in pregnancy; do **not** use in mouth (risk of choking); also **special care** in infants or young children

Side-effects include confusion, convulsions, respiratory depression, and cardiac depressant effects; allergic reactions (rarely anaphylaxis)

Administration see under preparations

◢*Prescribe as:*

Lidocaine Ointment

Ointment, lidocaine hydrochloride 5% in a water-miscible basis. Net price 15 g = £6.18.

Administration sore nipples from breast-feeding, apply using gauze and wash off immediately before feed

Lidocaine and Chlorhexidine Gel

Gel in disposable syringe, lidocaine hydrochloride 2%, chlorhexidine gluconate solution 0.25%, in a sterile lubricant basis in disposable syringe. Net price 6-mL syringe = 23p, 11-mL syringe = 14p. *Proprietary product: Instillagel* (6 mL, 11 mL)

Administration into urethra, 6–11 mL

---

1. Nurse prescribers should prescribe packs containing no more than **32 tablets**, a max. of **3** packs of 32 tablets may be prescribed on each occasion: [PoM] but may be sold to the public under certain circumstances—for details see *Medicines, Ethics and Practice*, London, Pharmaceutical Press (always consult latest edition)

Prevention of neural tube defects

Corresponds to BNF section 9.1.2.

Prevention of neural tube defects

Folic acid supplements taken before and during pregnancy can reduce the occurrence of neural tube defects. The risk of a neural tube defect occurring in a child should be assessed and folic acid given as follows:

> Women at a low risk of conceiving a child with a neural tube defect should be advised to take folic acid as a medicinal or food supplement at a dose of 400 micrograms daily before conception and until week 12 of pregnancy. Women who have not been taking folic acid and who suspect they are pregnant should start at once and continue until week 12 of pregnancy.

> Couples are at a high risk of conceiving a child with a neural tube defect if either partner has a neural tube defect (or either partner has a family history of neural tube defects), if they have had a previous pregnancy affected by a neural tube defect, or if the woman has coeliac disease (or other malabsorption state), diabetes mellitus, sickle-cell anaemia, or is taking antiepileptic medicines (see also BNF section 4.8.1).

> Women in the high-risk group who wish to become pregnant (or who are at risk of becoming pregnant) should be referred to a doctor because a higher dose of folic acid is appropriate.

Folic acid 400 microgram tablets are available for prescription. *Healthy Start Vitamins for Women* (containing folic acid, ascorbic acid, and vitamin D) are available for pregnant women through the Healthy Start Scheme (but not on prescription)—see BNF section 9.6.1 and information for healthcare professionals at www.healthystart.nhs.uk. Vitamins for children are also available through the scheme.

 FOLIC ACID

Indications prevention of neural tube defects, see notes above

Cautions interactions: see BNF Appendix 1 (folates)

Side-effects *rarely* gastro-intestinal disturbances

Dose

● See notes above

◢*Prescribe as:*

¹**Folic Acid Tablets, 400 micrograms**

Tablets, folic acid 400 micrograms, net price 90-tab pack = £2.71. *Proprietary product: Preconceive and possibly others*

――――――――――――――――――――
1. Can be sold to the public provided daily doses do not exceed 500 micrograms

Nicotine replacement therapy

Corresponds to BNF section 4.10.2

Smoking cessation interventions are a cost-effective way of reducing ill health and prolonging life. Smokers should be advised to stop and offered help if interested in doing so, with follow-up where appropriate. If possible, smokers should have access to smoking cessation services for behavioural support.

Therapy to aid smoking cessation is chosen according to the smoker's preferences, availability of counselling and support, previous experience of smoking-cessation aids, contra-indications and adverse effects of the products.

Nicotine replacement therapy is an effective aid to smoking cessation. The use of nicotine replacement preparations in an individual who is already accustomed to nicotine introduces few new risks and is widely accepted that there are no circumstances in which it is safer to smoke than to use nicotine replacement therapy.

Nicotine replacement therapy can be used in place of cigarettes after abrupt cessation of smoking, or alternatively to reduce the amount of cigarettes used in advance of making a quit attempt. Nicotine replacement therapy can also be used to minimise passive smoking, and to treat cravings and reduce compensatory smoking after enforced abstinence in smoke-free environments. Smokers who find it difficult to achieve abstinence should consult a healthcare professional for advice.

Choice   Nicotine patches are a prolonged-release formulation and are applied for 16 hours (with the patch removed overnight) or for 24 hours. If patients experience strong cravings for cigarettes on waking, a 24-hour patch may be more suitable. Immediate-release nicotine preparations (gum, lozenges, sublingual tablets, inhalator, nasal spray, and oral spray) are used whenever the urge to smoke occurs or to prevent cravings.

The choice of nicotine replacement preparation depends largely on patient preference, and should take into account what preparations, if any, have been tried before. Patients with a high level of nicotine dependence, or who have failed with nicotine replacement therapy previously, may benefit from using a combination of an immediate-release preparation and patches to achieve abstinence.

All preparations are licensed for adults and children over 12 years (with the exception of *Nicotinell®* lozenges which are licensed for children under 18 years only when recommended by a doctor).

Cautions   Most warnings for nicotine replacement therapy also apply to continued cigarette smoking, but the risk of continued smoking outweighs any risks of using nicotine preparations. Nicotine replacement therapy should be used with caution in haemodynamically unstable patients hospitalised with severe arrhythmias, myocardial infarction, or cerebrovascular accident, and in patients with phaeochromocytoma or uncontrolled hyperthyroidism. Care is also needed in patients with diabetes mellitus—blood-glucose concentration should be monitored closely when initiating treatment.

Specific cautions for individual preparations are usually related to the local effect of nicotine. *Oral preparations* should be used with caution in patients with oesophagitis, gastritis, or peptic ulcers because swallowed nicotine can aggravate these conditions. The *gum* may also stick to and damage dentures. Acidic beverages, such as coffee or fruit juice, may decrease the absorption of nicotine through the buccal mucosa and should be avoided for 15 minutes before the use of oral nicotine replacement therapy. Care should be taken with the *inhalation cartridges* in patients with obstructive lung disease, chronic throat disease, or bronchospastic disease. The *nasal spray* can cause worsening of bronchial asthma. *Patches* should not be placed on broken skin and should be used with caution in patients with skin disorders.

Hepatic impairment   Nicotine replacement therapy should be used with caution in moderate to severe hepatic impairment.

Renal impairment   Nicotine replacement therapy should be used with caution in severe renal impairment.

Pregnancy   The use of nicotine replacement therapy in pregnancy is preferable to the continuation of smoking, but should be used only if smoking cessation without nicotine replacement fails. Intermittent therapy is preferable to patches but avoid liquorice-flavoured nicotine products. Patches are useful, however, if the patient is experiencing pregnancy-related nausea and vomiting. If patches are used, they should be removed before bed.

Breast-feeding   Nicotine is present in milk; however, the amount to which the infant is exposed is small and less hazardous than second-hand smoke. Intermittent therapy is preferred.

Side-effects   Some systemic effects occur on initiation of therapy, particularly if the patient is using high-strength preparations; however, the patient may confuse side-effects of the nicotine-replacement preparation with nicotine withdrawal symptoms. Common symptoms of nicotine withdrawal include malaise, headache, dizziness, sleep disturbance, coughing, influenza-like symptoms, depression, irritability, increased appetite, weight gain, restlessness, anxiety, drowsiness, aphthous ulcers, decreased heart rate, and impaired concentration.

Mild local reactions at the beginning of treatment are common because of the irritant effect of nicotine. *Oral preparations* and *inhalation cartridges* can cause irritation of the throat, *gum*, *lozenges*, and *oral spray* can cause increased salivation, and *patches* can cause minor skin irritation. The *nasal spray* commonly causes coughing, nasal irritation, epistaxis, sneezing, and watery eyes; the *oral spray* can cause watery eyes and blurred vision.

Gastro-intestinal disturbances are common and may be caused by swallowed nicotine. Nausea, vomiting, dyspepsia, and hiccup occur most frequently. Ulcerative stomatitis has also been reported. Dry mouth is a common side-effect of *lozenges*, *patches*, *oral spray*, and *sublingual tablets*. *Lozenges* cause diarrhoea, constipation, dysphagia, oesophagitis, gastritis, mouth ulcers, bloating, flatulence, and less commonly, taste disturbance, thirst, gingival bleeding, and halitosis. The *oral spray* may also cause abdominal pain, flatulence, and taste disturbance.

Palpitations may occur with nicotine replacement therapy and rarely *patches* and *oral spray* can cause arrhythmia. *Patches*, *lozenges*, and *oral spray* can cause chest pain. The *inhalator* can very rarely cause reversible atrial fibrillation.

Paraesthesia is a common side-effect of *oral spray*. Abnormal dreams can occur with *patches*; removal of the patch before bed may help. *Lozenges* and *oral spray* may cause rash and hot flushes. Sweating and myalgia can occur with *patches* and *oral spray*; the *patches* can also cause arthralgia.

Nicotine medicated chewing gum   Individuals who smoke fewer than 20 cigarettes each day should use 1 piece of 2-mg strength gum when the urge to smoke occurs or to prevent cravings; individuals who smoke more than 20 cigarettes each day or who require more than 15 pieces of 2-mg strength gum each day should use the 4-mg strength. Patients should not exceed 15 pieces of 4-mg strength gum daily. If attempting smoking cessation, treatment should continue for 3 months before reducing the dose.

Administration   Chew the gum until the taste becomes strong, then rest it between the cheek and gum; when the taste starts to fade, repeat this process. One piece of gum lasts for approximately 30 minutes.

Nicotine inhalation cartridge   The cartridges can be used when the urge to smoke occurs or to prevent cravings. Patients should not exceed 12 cartridges of the 10 mg strength daily, or 6 cartridges of the 15 mg strength daily.

Administration   Insert the cartridge into the device and draw in air through the mouthpiece; each session can last for approximately 5 minutes. The amount of nicotine from 1 puff of the cartridge is less than that from a cigarette, therefore it is necessary to inhale more often than when smoking a cigarette. A single 10 mg cartridge lasts for approximately 20 minutes of intense use; a single 15 mg cartridge lasts for approximately 40 minutes of intense use.

Nicotine lozenge   One lozenge should be used every 1–2 hours when the urge to smoke occurs. Individuals who smoke less than 20 cigarettes each day should usually use the lower-strength lozenges; individuals who smoke more than 20 cigarettes each day and those who fail to stop smoking with the low-strength lozenges should use the higher-strength lozenges. Patients should not exceed 15 lozenges daily. If attempting smoking cessation, treatment should continue for 6–12 weeks before attempting a reduction in dose.

Administration   Slowly allow each lozenge to dissolve in the mouth; periodically move the lozenge from one side of the mouth to the other. Lozenges last for 10–30 minutes, depending on their size.

Nicotine sublingual tablets   Individuals who smoke fewer than 20 cigarettes each day should initially use 1 tablet each hour, increased to 2 tablets each hour if necessary; individuals who smoke more than 20 cigarettes each day should use 2 tablets each hour. Patients should not exceed 40 tablets daily. If attempting smoking cessation, treatment should continue for up to 3 months before reducing the dose.

Administration   Each tablet should be placed under the tongue and allowed to dissolve.

Nicotine oral spray   Patients can use 1–2 sprays in the mouth when the urge to smoke occurs or to prevent cravings. Individuals should not exceed 2 sprays per episode (up to 4 sprays every hour), and a maximum of 64 sprays daily.

Administration The oral spray should be released into the mouth, holding the spray as close to the mouth as possible and avoiding the lips. The patient should not inhale while spraying and avoid swallowing for a few seconds after use.

Note If using the oral spray for the first time, or if unit not used for 2 or more days, prime the unit before administration.

Nicotine nasal spray Patients can use 1 spray in each nostril when the urge to smoke occurs, up to twice every hour for 16 hours daily (maximum 64 sprays daily). If attempting smoking cessation, treatment should continue for 8 weeks before reducing the dose.

Administration Initially 1 spray should be used in both nostrils but when withdrawing from therapy, the dose can be gradually reduced to 1 spray in 1 nostril.

Nicotine transdermal patches As a general guide for smoking cessation, individuals who smoke more than 10 cigarettes daily should apply a high-strength patch daily for 6–8 weeks, followed by the medium-strength patch for 2 weeks, and then the low-strength patch for the final 2 weeks; individuals who smoke fewer than 10 cigarettes daily can usually start with the medium-strength patch for 6–8 weeks, followed by the low-strength patch for 2–4 weeks. A slower titration schedule can be used in patients who are not ready to quit but want to reduce cigarette consumption before a quit attempt.

If abstinence is not achieved, or if withdrawal symptoms are experienced, the strength of the patch used should be maintained or increased until the patient is stabilised. Patients using the high-strength patch who experience excessive side-effects, that do not resolve within a few days, should change to a medium-strength patch for the remainder of the initial period and then use the low-strength patch for 2–4 weeks.

Administration Patches should be applied on waking to dry, non-hairy skin on the hip, trunk, or upper arm and held in position for 10–20 seconds to ensure adhesion; place next patch on a different area and avoid using the same site for several days.

> Cross-references to the BNF are provided but nurse prescribers may only prescribe those items that are listed on the Nurse Prescribers' List.

◢ NICOTINE

Indications see notes above

Cautions see notes above; **interactions**: see BNF Appendix 1 (nicotine)

Hepatic impairment see notes above

Renal impairment see notes above

Pregnancy see notes above

Breast-feeding see notes above

Side-effects see notes above

Dose

• See notes above

◢*Prescribe as:*

[1]Nicotine Inhalation Cartridge for Oromucosal Use

Cartridge (for oromucosal use), nicotine 10 mg, net price 6-cartridge (starter) pack = £4.46, 42-cartridge (refill) pack = £14.65; 15 mg, net price 4-cartridge pack = £4.14, 20-cartridge pack = £14.67, 36-cartridge pack = £22.33. *Proprietary products: NicAssist Inhalator, Nicorette Inhalator*

Nicotine Lozenge

Lozenge, sugar-free, nicotine (as bitartrate) 1 mg, net price pack of 12 = £1.71, pack of 36 = £4.27, pack of 96 = £9.12; 2 mg, pack of 12 = £1.99, pack of 24 =£2.55, pack of 36 = £4.95, pack of 96 = £8.29 (*proprietary products: Nicorette Mint Lozenge, Nicotinell Mint Lozenge*) *or* nicotine (as resinate) 1.5 mg, net price pack of 20 = £3.18, pack of 60 = £8.93; 2 mg, pack of 36 = £5.12, pack of 72 = £9.97; 4 mg pack of 20 = £3.18, pack of 36 = £5.12, pack of 60 = £8.93, pack of 72 = £9.97 (*proprietary products: NiQuitin Lozenge, NiQuitin Minis, NiQuitin Pre-quit*)

Excipients include aspartame (BNF section 9.4.1)

Nicotine Sublingual Tablets

Sublingual tablet, nicotine (as a cyclodextrin complex) 2 mg, net price starter pack of 2 × 15-tablet discs with dispenser = £4.83, refill pack of 100 = £13.12. *Proprietary products: NicAssist Microtab, Nicorette Microtab*

Excipients lemon flavour includes aspartame (BNF section 9.4.1)

Nicotine Medicated Chewing Gum

Chewing gum, sugar-free, nicotine 2 mg, net price pack of 12 = £1.71, pack of 24 = £2.85, pack of 96 = £8.55; 4 mg, net price pack of 12 = £1.71, pack of 24 = £2.85, pack of 96 = £8.55 (*proprietary product: NiQuitin Gum*), *or* nicotine (as polacrilin complex) 2 mg, net price pack of 12 = £1.71, pack of 24 = £3.01, pack of 72 = £6.69, pack of 96 = £8.26, pack of 204 = £14.23; 4 mg, net price pack of 12 = £1.70, pack of 24 = £3.30, pack of 72 = £8.29, pack of 96 = £10.26 (*proprietary product: Nicotinell Gum*), *or* nicotine (as resin) 2 mg, net price pack of 30 = £3.25, pack of 105 = £9.27, pack of 210 = £14.82; 4 mg, net price pack of 30 = £3.99, pack of 105 = £11.28, pack of 210 = £18.24 (*proprietary products: NicAssist Gum, Nicorette Gum*)

Note Available in various flavours

Nicotine Nasal Spray

Nasal spray, nicotine 500 micrograms/metered spray, net price 200-spray unit = £13.40. *Proprietary products: NicAssist Nasal Spray, Nicorette Nasal Spray*

Nicotine Oral Spray

Oral spray, nicotine 1 mg/metered dose, net price 150-dose pack = £12.12, 2 × 150-dose pack = £19.14. *Proprietary product: Nicorette QuickMist Mouthspray*

Note contains <100 mg ethanol per dose

---

1. For use with an inhalation mouthpiece; starter pack contains 6 cartridges with inhalator device and holder, refill pack contains 42 cartridges with inhalator device

[1]**Nicotine Transdermal Patches**

Patches, self-adhesive, releasing in each 16 hours, nicotine approx. 5 mg, 10 mg, or 15 mg (*proprietary product: NicAssist Patch, Nicorette Patch*), *or* releasing in 16 hours approx. 10 mg, 15 mg, or 25 mg (*proprietary products: NicAssist Translucent Patch, Nicorette Invisi Patch*), *or* releasing in each 24 hours nicotine approx. 7 mg, 14 mg, or 21 mg (*proprietary products: Nicotinell TTS, NiQuitin, NiQuitin Clear*)

Note for pack sizes and prices, see individual products in BNF section 4.10

Drugs for the mouth

Corresponds to BNF sections 12.3.2, 12.3.1, 12.3.4 and 12.3.5

Candida albicans may cause thrush and other forms of stomatitis which sometimes follow the use of inhaled corticosteroids, broad-spectrum antibacterials or cytotoxics; any underlying cause should be appropriately managed. Antifungal treatment may be required; when thrush is associated with corticosteroid inhalers, rinsing the mouth with water (or cleaning a child's teeth) immediately after using the inhaler may avoid the problem. Infants may develop thrush which responds to use of an antifungal mouth preparation.

Patients with denture stomatitis may also respond to the use of an antifungal mouth preparation. They should be instructed to cleanse their dentures thoroughly to prevent reinfection; ideally they should leave their dentures out as often as possible during the treatment period. Proper dental appraisal may be necessary.

Oral antifungal drugs

Miconazole and **nystatin** are suitable for the treatment of oral thrush. Topical therapy may not be adequate in immunocompromised patients and an oral triazole antifungal is preferred; Community Practitioner nurse prescribers should refer the patient to a doctor or appropriate independent prescriber.

MICONAZOLE

Indications prevention and treatment of oral fungal infections

Cautions interactions: see BNF Appendix 1 (antifungals, imidazole); oral gel may be absorbed enough for interactions to occur after application to the oral mucosa

Contra-indications acute porphyria (BNF section 9.8.2); impaired swallowing reflex in infants; first 6 months of life of an infant born preterm

Hepatic impairment avoid

Pregnancy manufacturer advises avoid if possible—toxicity at high doses in *animal* studies

Breast-feeding manufacturer advises caution—no information available

Side-effects nausea, vomiting; rash; *very rarely* diarrhoea (usually on long-term treatment), hepatitis, toxic epidermal necrolysis, and Stevens-Johnson syndrome

Dose
- See under preparation

◢*Prescribe as:*

[2]**Miconazole Oromucosal Gel** PoM

Oral gel, sugar-free, orange-flavoured, miconazole 24 mg/mL (20 mg/g). Net price 15-g tube = £2.97, 80-g tube = £4.38. *Proprietary product: Daktarin Oral Gel*

Dose place 5–10 mL in the mouth after food 4 times daily; retain near oral lesions before swallowing; CHILD 4 months–2 years 2.5 mL twice daily, smeared around the inside of the mouth; 2–6 years 5 mL twice daily, retained near lesions before swallowing; over 6 years 5 mL 4 times daily, retained near lesions before swallowing; treatment continued for 48 hours after lesions have healed

Localised lesions, ADULT and CHILD over 2 years, smear small

---

amount of gel on affected area with clean finger 4 times daily for 5–7 days (dentures should be removed at night and brushed with gel); treatment continued for 48 hours after lesions have healed (prescribe 15-g tube)

Note Not licensed for use in children under 4 months of age or during first 6 months of life of an infant born preterm

NYSTATIN

Indications oral and perioral fungal infections

Side-effects oral irritation and sensitisation, nausea reported

Dose
- See under preparation, below

◢*Prescribe as:*

Nystatin Oral Suspension PoM
Oral suspension, nystatin 100 000 units/mL. Net price 30 mL = £1.80

Dose ADULT and CHILD over 1 month, place 1 mL in the mouth after food and retain near the lesions 4 times daily, usually for 7 days (continued for 48 hours after lesions have resolved); NEONATE [unlicensed], place 1 mL in the mouth 4 times daily after feeds, usually for 7 days (continued for 48 hours after lesions have healed)

Note Not licensed for treating candidiasis in NEONATE under 1 month but the Department of Health has advised that a Community Practitioner Nurse Prescriber may prescribe nystatin oral suspension for a NEONATE, at the dose stated above, provided that there is a clear diagnosis of oral thrush. The nurse prescriber must only prescribe within their own competence and must accept clinical and medicolegal responsibility for prescribing

Thymol

Mouthwashes have a mechanical cleansing action. **Mouthwash solution-tablets** may contain thymol as well as an antimicrobial; they are used to remove unpleasant tastes.

THYMOL

Indications oral hygiene, see notes above

Dose
- See under preparation, below

◢*Prescribe as:*

Mouthwash Solution-tablets
Tablets, may contain antimicrobial, colouring, and flavouring agents in a suitable soluble effervescent basis to make a mouthwash. Net price 100-tab pack = £15.09

Dose dissolve 1 tablet in a glass of warm water and rinse
Note Mouthwash Solution-tablets may contain ingredients such as thymol

Drugs for oral ulceration and inflammation

Choline salicylate dental gel has some analgesic action and may provide relief for recurrent mouth ulcers, but excessive application or confinement under a denture irritates the mucosa and can itself cause ulceration. Choline salicylate dental gel should no longer be used for teething or in children under 16 years, because of the theoretical risk of Reye's syndrome.

> Patients with an unexplained mouth ulcer of more than 3 weeks' duration require urgent referral to exclude oral cancer.

SALICYLATES

Indications mild oral and perioral lesions

Cautions not to be applied to dentures—leave at least 30 minutes before re-insertion of dentures; frequent application, especially in children, may give rise to salicylate poisoning

Contra-indications children under 16 years
Reye's syndrome The CHM has advised (April 2009) that topical oral pain relief products containing salicylate salts should not be used in children under 16 years, as a cautionary measure due to the theoretical risk of Reye's syndrome

Dose
- ADULT and CHILD over 16 years, apply $\frac{1}{2}$-inch of gel with gentle massage not more often than every 3 hours

◢*Prescribe as:*

Choline Salicylate Dental Gel
Oral gel, choline salicylate 8.7% in a flavoured gel basis, net price 15 g = £2.13. *Proprietary product: Bonjela* (sugar-free)

Treatment of dry mouth

Dry mouth may be relieved in many patients by simple measures such as frequent sips of cool drinks or sucking pieces of ice or sugar-free fruit pastilles. Sugar-free chewing gum stimulates salivation in patients with residual salivary function.

Saliva stimulating tablets may be prescribed for dry mouth in patients with salivary gland impairment (and patent salivary ducts).

◢*Prescribe as:*

Saliva Stimulating Tablets
Tablets, sugar-free, citric acid, malic acid and other ingredients in a sorbitol base, net price 100-tab pack = £4.86. *Proprietary product: SST tablets*

Dose symptomatic treatment of dry mouth in patients with impaired salivary gland function and patent salivary ducts, allow 1 tablet to dissolve slowly in the mouth when required

Removal of earwax

Corresponds to BNF section 12.1.3

Wax is a normal bodily secretion which provides a protective film on the meatal skin and need only be removed if it causes hearing loss or interferes with a proper view of the ear drum.

Wax can be softened with simple remedies such as **olive oil** ear drops or **almond oil** ear drops. **Sodium bicarbonate** ear drops are also effective but may cause dryness of the ear canal. If the wax is hard and impacted, the drops may be used twice daily for several days and this may reduce the need for mechanical removal of the wax. The patient should lie with the affected ear uppermost for 5 to 10 minutes after a generous amount of the softening remedy has been introduced into the ear.

If necessary, wax may be removed by irrigation with water (warmed to body temperature). Ear irrigation is generally best avoided in young children, in patients unable to co-operate with the procedure, in those with otitis media in the last six weeks, in otitis externa, in patients with cleft palate, a history of ear drum perforation, or previous ear surgery. A person who has hearing only in one ear should not have that ear irrigated because even a very slight risk of damage is unacceptable in this situation.

> Cross references to the BNF are provided but nurse prescribers may only prescribe those items that are listed on the Nurse Prescribers' List.

◢*Prescribe as:*

Almond Oil Ear Drops
Ear drops, almond oil in a suitable container
Administration allow to warm to room temperature and use as indicated above
Note Do not heat

Olive Oil Ear Drops
Ear drops, olive oil in a suitable container
Administration allow to warm to room temperature and use as indicated above
Note Do not heat

Sodium Bicarbonate Ear Drops
Ear drops, sodium bicarbonate 5%. Net price 10 mL = £1.25
Administration allow to warm to room temperature and use as indicated above

Drugs for threadworms

Corresponds to BNF section 5.5.1.

Anthelmintics are effective for threadworm infections (enterobiasis) but their use needs to be combined with hygiene measures to break the cycle of auto-infection. Threadworms are highly infectious therefore all members of the family need to be treated at the same time.

Adult threadworms do not live for longer than 6 weeks; eggs need to be swallowed and subjected to the action of digestive juices in the upper intestinal tract for the development of the worms. Direct multiplication of worms does not take place in the large bowel. Adult female worms lay eggs on the perianal skin, which causes *pruritus*. Scratching the area leads to eggs being transmitted on fingers to the mouth, often via food eaten with unwashed hands. It is therefore important to advise patients to wash their hands and scrub their nails before each meal and after each visit to the toilet. A bath taken immediately after rising will remove eggs laid during the night. Advice for patients is included in the packaging of most preparations, but it is useful to reinforce this advice verbally.

> Mebendazole and piperazine are also prescribed for other infections (e.g. roundworms). Community Practitioner nurse prescribers should, however, prescribe them for threadworm infection **only.**

Mebendazole

Mebendazole is the drug of choice for patients over 2 years of age with threadworms. It is given as a single dose but as reinfection is very common, a second dose may be given after 2 weeks.

◢ MEBENDAZOLE

Indications threadworm infection; other infections, on doctor's prescription only
Cautions interactions: BNF Appendix 1 (mebendazole)
Pregnancy manufacturer advises toxicity in *animal* studies—see below for warnings in packs
Breast-feeding amount too small to be harmful but manufacturer advises avoid
Side-effects abdominal pain; *less commonly* diarrhoea, flatulence; *rarely* hepatitis, convulsions, dizziness, neutropenia, urticaria, alopecia, rash (including Stevens-Johnson syndrome and toxic epidermal necrolysis)
Dose
● Threadworms, ADULT and CHILD over 2 years, 100 mg as a single dose; if reinfection occurs second dose may be needed after 2 weeks; CHILD under 2 years not recommended

◢*Prescribe as:*

[1]**Mebendazole Tablets 100 mg** PoM
Tablets, chewable, mebendazole 100 mg. Net price 6-tab pack = £1.36.
Note The package insert includes the information that the

---

1. Packs containing no more than 800 mg and labelled to show a max. single dose of 100 mg are on sale to the public for the treatment of threadworm infection in adults and children over 2 years

tablets are not suitable for women known to be pregnant or for children under 2 years

¹Mebendazole Oral Suspension 100 mg/5 mL PoM
Oral Suspension, mebendazole 100 mg/5 mL. Net price 30 mL = £1.59. *Proprietary product: Vermox*
Note The package insert includes the information that the suspension is not suitable for women known to be pregnant or for children under 2 years

Piperazine

Piperazine is available in combination with sennosides; 2 doses are given for threadworm infection with an interval of 2 weeks between them.

◼ PIPERAZINE

Indications threadworm infection; other infections, on doctor's prescription only

Cautions epilepsy—see below for warnings in packs

Hepatic impairment manufacturer advises avoid

Renal impairment use with caution; avoid in severe renal impairment; risk of neurotoxicity

Pregnancy not known to be harmful but manufacturer advises avoid in first trimester—see below for warnings in packs

Breast-feeding present in milk—manufacturer advises avoid breast-feeding for 8 hours after dose (express and discard milk during this time)

Side-effects nausea, vomiting, colic, diarrhoea; allergic reactions including urticaria, bronchospasm, and rare reports of arthralgia, fever, Stevens-Johnson syndrome and angioedema; rarely dizziness, muscular incoordination ('worm wobble'); drowsiness, nystagmus, vertigo, blurred vision, confusion and clonic contractions in patients with neurological or renal abnormalities

Dose
• Threadworms, see under preparation, below

◢*Prescribe as:*

For cautions, contra-indications, and side-effects of Senna, see p. 8

Piperazine and Senna Powder
Oral powder, piperazine phosphate 4 g, total sennosides (calculated as sennoside B) 15.3 mg/sachet. Net price 2-dose sachet pack = £1.98. *Proprietary product: Pripsen*
Dose stirred into a small glass of milk or water and drunk immediately, ADULT and CHILD over 6 years, content of 1 sachet as a single dose (bedtime in adults or morning in children), repeated after 14 days; CHILD 3 months–1 year, 1 level 2.5-mL spoonful in the morning, repeated after 14 days; CHILD 1–6 years, 1 level 5-mL spoonful in the morning, repeated after 14 days
Cautionary label added by pharmacist: dissolve or mix with water before taking
Note For children under 10 years, only one dual-dose treatment should be given in any 28-day period without medical advice. Packs on sale to the public carry a warning to avoid in epilepsy, in liver or kidney disease, and to seek medical advice in pregnancy

---

1. Packs containing no more than 800 mg and labelled to show a max. single dose of 100 mg are on sale to the public for the treatment of threadworm infection in adults and children over 2 years

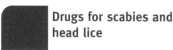

Drugs for scabies and head lice

Corresponds to BNF section 13.10.4

Scabies

Permethrin is used for the treatment of *scabies* (*Sarcoptes scabiei*); **malathion** can be used if permethrin is not appropriate.

Although acaricides have traditionally been applied after a hot bath, this is **not** necessary and there is even evidence that a hot bath may increase absorption into the blood, removing them from their site of action on the skin.

All members of the affected household should be treated simultaneously. Treatment should be applied to the whole body including the scalp, neck, face, and ears. Particular attention should be paid to the webs of the fingers and toes, and lotion brushed under the ends of the nails. It is now recommended that malathion and permethrin should be applied twice, one week apart. Patients with hyperkeratotic (crusted or 'Norwegian') scabies may require 2 or 3 applications of acaricide on consecutive days to ensure that enough penetrates the skin crusts to kill all the mites.

It is important to warn users to reapply treatment to the hands if they are washed.

The itch of scabies persists for some weeks after the infestation has been eliminated and antipruritic treatment may be required. Application of **crotamiton** (p. 25) can be used to control itching after treatment with more effective acaricides, but caution is necessary if the skin is excoriated.

> Cross references to the BNF are provided but nurse prescribers may only prescribe those items that are listed on the Nurse Prescribers' List.

Head lice

Dimeticone is effective against head lice (*Pediculus humanus capitis*) and acts on the surface of the organism. Malathion, an organophosphorus insecticide, is an alternative, but resistance has been reported.

Head lice infestation (pediculosis) should be treated with lotion or liquid formulations only if live lice are present. Shampoos are diluted too much in use to be effective. A contact time of 8–12 hours or overnight treatment is recommended for lotions and liquids. A 2-hour treatment is not sufficient to kill eggs.

In general, a course of treatment for head lice should be 2 applications of product 7 days apart to kill lice emerging from any eggs that survive the first application. All affected household members should be treated simultaneously.

Wet combing methods Head lice may be mechanically removed by combing wet hair meticulously with a plastic detection comb (probably for at least 30 minutes each time) over the whole scalp at 4-day intervals for a minimum of 2 weeks, and continued until no lice are found on 3 consecutive sessions; hair conditioner can be used to facilitate the process. Combing devices and topical solutions to aid the removal of head lice are available and some are prescribable on the NHS, including *Bug Buster kit*, *Full Marks Solution*, *Linicin Lotion 15 mins*, *Nitcomb-M2*, *Nitcomb-S1*, *Nitlotion*, *Nitty Gritty NitFree*, *NYDA*, and *Portia Head Lice Comb* (consult Drug Tariff—see Appliances and Reagents (p. 5) for links to online Drug Tariffs).

> Not all preparations included here are licensed for *crab lice* therefore advice on crab lice has not been included

> Individuals can rarely react to certain ingredients in preparations applied to the skin. Special care is required when prescribing skin and scalp products for these individuals—see BNF section 13.1.3. Excipients associated with sensitisation are shown under individual product entries

Dimeticone

Dimeticone coats head lice and interferes with water balance in lice by preventing the excretion of water; it is less active against eggs and treatment should be repeated after 7 days.

▌ DIMETICONE

Indications head lice

Cautions avoid contact with eyes; children under 6 months, medical supervision required

Side-effects skin irritation

Administration rub into dry hair and scalp, allow to dry naturally, shampoo after minimum 8 hours (or overnight); repeat application after 7 days

◢*Prescribe as:*

Dimeticone Lotion 4%
Lotion, dimeticone 4%, net price 50 mL = £2.98, 120-mL spray pack = £7.13, 150 mL = £6.92. *Proprietary product: Hedrin*
Note Patients should be told to keep hair away from fire and flames during treatment

Malathion

Malathion is recommended for *scabies* and *head lice* (for details see notes above).

The risk of systemic effects associated with 1–2 applications of malathion is considered to be very low; however applications of lotions repeated at intervals of less than 1 week *or* application for more than 3 consecutive weeks should be **avoided** since the likelihood of eradication of lice is not increased.

▌ MALATHION

Indications scabies, head lice

Cautions avoid contact with eyes; do not use on broken or secondarily infected skin; do not use more than once a week for 3 consecutive weeks; use in children under 6 months on doctor's advice only

Side-effects skin irritation and hypersensitivity reactions; chemical burns also reported

Administration head lice, rub into dry hair and scalp, allow to dry naturally, remove by washing 12 hours later (see also notes above); repeat application after 7 days

Scabies, apply over whole body, wash off after 24 hours; if hands are washed with soap within 24 hours, they should be retreated; see also notes above; repeat application after 7 days
Note For scabies, manufacturer recommends application to the body but not necessarily to the head and neck. However, application should be extended to the scalp, neck, face, and ears.

◢*Prescribe as:*

Malathion Aqueous Lotion 0.5%
Aqueous lotion, malathion 0.5% in an aqueous basis. *Proprietary products: Derbac-M Liquid* (net price 50 mL = £2.37, 200 mL = £5.93)
Excipients include cetostearyl alcohol, fragrance, hydroxybenzoates (parabens)

Permethrin

Permethrin is effective for *scabies* (for details see notes above). Permethrin is active against *head lice* but the formulation and licensed methods of application of the current products make them unsuitable for the treatment of head lice.

▌ PERMETHRIN

Indications scabies

Cautions avoid contact with eyes; do not use on broken or secondarily infected skin; use for scabies in children under 2 years on doctor's advice only

Side-effects pruritus, erythema, and stinging; rarely rashes and oedema

Administration scabies, apply over whole body and wash off after 8–12 hours; CHILD (see also Cautions above) apply over whole body including face, neck, scalp, and ears; cream should be reapplied to hands if they are washed with soap and water within 8 hours of application (see notes above); repeat application after 7 days
Note Manufacturer recommends application to the body but to exclude the head and neck. However, application should be extended to the scalp, neck, face, and ears.
Larger patients may require up to two 30-g packs for adequate treatment

◢*Prescribe as:*

Permethrin Cream 5%
Cream, permethrin 5%. Net price 30 g = £5.71. *Proprietary product: Lyclear Dermal Cream*
Excipients may include butylated hydroxytoluene, wool fat derivative

Skin preparations

Emollients

Corresponds to BNF section 13.2.1 and 13.2.1.1.

Emollients soothe, smooth and hydrate the skin and are indicated for all dry or scaling disorders. Their effects are short-lived and they should be applied frequently even after improvement occurs. They are useful in dry and eczematous disorders, and to a lesser extent in psoriasis. The choice of an appropriate emollient will often depend on the severity of the condition, patient preference and site of application. Emollient preparations contained in tubs should be removed with a clean spoon or spatula to reduce bacterial contamination of the emollient. Emollients should be applied in the direction of hair growth to reduce the risk of folliculitis. Ointments may exacerbate acne and folliculitis. Some ingredients may occasionally cause sensitisation (BNF section 13.1.3) and this should be suspected if an eczematous reaction occurs. The use of aqueous cream as a leave-on emollient may increase the risk of skin reactions, particularly in eczema.

> **Fire hazard with paraffin-based emollients**
> Emulsifying ointment *or* 50% Liquid Paraffin and 50% White Soft Paraffin Ointment in contact with dressings and clothing is easily ignited by a naked flame. The risk will be greater when these preparations are applied to large areas of the body, and clothing or dressings become soaked with the ointment. Patients should be told to keep away from fire or flames, and not to smoke when using these preparations. The risk of fire should be considered when using large quantities of any paraffin-based emollient.

Preparations such as **aqueous cream** and **emulsifying ointment** can be used as soap substitutes for hand washing and in the bath; the preparation is rubbed on the skin before rinsing off completely. The addition of a bath oil may also be helpful. Several proprietary emollient bath additives and shower preparations are available (see below). Emollient bath and shower preparations make skin and surfaces slippery—particular care is needed when bathing.

Urea is a keratin softener and hydrating agent used in the treatment of dry, scaling conditions (including ichthyosis) and may be useful in elderly patients.

> Individuals can rarely react to certain ingredients in preparations applied to the skin. Special care is required when prescribing skin and scalp products for these individuals—see BNF section 13.1.3. Excipients associated with sensitisation are shown under individual product entries

EMOLLIENTS

◢ *Prescribe as:*

Emulsifying Ointment
Ointment, emulsifying wax 30%, white soft paraffin 50%, liquid paraffin 20%, net price 500 g = £2.49
Excipients include cetostearyl alcohol

Hydrous Ointment
(Also known as Oily Cream)
Ointment, dried magnesium sulfate 0.5%, phenoxyethanol 1%, wool alcohols ointment 50% in freshly boiled and cooled purified water, net price 500 g = £3.91

Liquid and White Soft Paraffin Ointment
Ointment, liquid paraffin 50%, white soft paraffin 50%, net price 500 g = £2.36

Paraffin, White Soft
White petroleum jelly, net price 100 g = 50p

Paraffin, Yellow Soft
Yellow petroleum jelly, net price 100 g = 54p

◢ **Proprietary emollients,** *prescribe as:*

Aquamax® (Dermato Logical)
Cream, light liquid paraffin 8%, white soft paraffin 20%, phenoxyethanol 1%, net price 30 g = 99p, 100 g = £1.89, 500 g = £3.99
Excipients include cetostearyl alcohol, polysorbate 60
For dry skin conditions

Aquamol® (Thornton & Ross)
Cream, containing liquid paraffin, white soft paraffin, net price 50 g = £1.22, 500-g pump pack = £6.40
Excipients include cetostearyl alcohol, chlorocresol
For dry skin conditions

Cetraben® Emollient Cream (Genus)
Cream, white soft paraffin 13.2%, light liquid paraffin 10.5%, net price 50-g pump pack = £1.40, 150-g pump pack = £3.98, 500-g pump pack = £5.99, 1.05-kg pump pack = £11.62
Excipients include cetostearyl alcohol, hydroxybenzoates (parabens)
For inflamed, damaged, dry or chapped skin including eczema

Dermamist® (Alliance)
Spray application, white soft paraffin 10% in a basis containing liquid paraffin, fractionated coconut oil, net price 250-mL pressurised aerosol unit = £5.97
For dry skin conditions including eczema, ichthyosis, pruritus of the elderly
Cautions flammable

Diprobase® Cream (Schering-Plough)
Cream, cetomacrogol 2.25%, cetostearyl alcohol 7.2%, liquid paraffin 6%, white soft paraffin 15%, water-miscible basis, net price 50 g = £1.28; 500-g pump pack = £6.32
Excipients include cetostearyl alcohol, chlorocresol
For dry skin conditions

Diprobase® Ointment (Schering-Plough)
Ointment, liquid paraffin 5%, white soft paraffin 95%, net price 50 g = £1.28, 500 g = £5.99
For dry skin conditions

Doublebase® (Dermal)
Gel, isopropyl myristate 15%, liquid paraffin 15%, net price 100 g = £2.65; 500 g = £5.83
For dry, chapped or itchy skin conditions

Doublebase® Dayleve Gel (Dermal)
Gel, isopropyl myristate 15%, liquid paraffin 15%, net price 100 g = £2.65, 500-g pump pack = £6.29
For dry, chapped, or itchy skin conditions

E45® Cream (Reckitt Benckiser)

Cream, light liquid paraffin 12.6%, white soft paraffin 14.5%, hypoallergenic anhydrous wool fat (hypoallergenic lanolin) 1% in self-emulsifying monostearin, net price 50 g = £1.61, 125 g = £2.90, 350 g = £4.85, 500-g pump pack = £5.62

Excipients include cetyl alcohol, hydroxybenzoates (parabens)

For dry skin conditions

Emollin® (C D Medical)

Spray, liquid paraffin 50%, white soft paraffin 50% in aerosol basis, net price 150 mL = £3.92, 240 mL = £6.26

For dry skin conditions

Epaderm® Cream (Mölnlycke)

Cream, yellow soft paraffin 15%, liquid paraffin 10%, emulsifying wax 5%, net price 50-g pump pack = £1.68, 500-g pump pack = £6.86

Excipients include cetostearyl alcohol, chlorocresol

For use as an emollient or soap substitute

Epaderm® Ointment (Mölnlycke)

Ointment, emulsifying wax 30%, yellow soft paraffin 30%, liquid paraffin 40%, net price 125 g = £3.85, 500 g = £6.53, 1 kg = £12.02

Excipients include cetostearyl alcohol

For use as an emollient or soap substitute

Hydromol® Cream (Alliance)

Cream, sodium pidolate 2.5%, liquid paraffin 13.8%, net price 50 g = £2.04, 100 g = £3.80, 500 g = £11.09

Excipients include cetostearyl alcohol, hydroxybenzoates (parabens)

For dry skin conditions

Hydromol® Ointment (Alliance)

Ointment, yellow soft paraffin 30%, emulsifying wax 30%, liquid paraffin 40%, net price 125 g = £2.84, 500 g = £4.82, 1 kg = £8.98

Excipients include cetostearyl alcohol

For use as an emollient, bath additive, or soap substitute

Lipobase® (Astellas)

Cream, fatty cream basis, net price 50 g = £1.46

Excipients include cetostearyl alcohol, hydroxybenzoates (parabens)

For dry skin conditions

Neutrogena® Norwegian Formula Dermatological Cream (J&J)

Cream, glycerol 40% in an emollient basis, net price 100 g = £6.32

Excipients include cetostearyl alcohol, hydroxybenzoates (parabens)

For dry skin conditions

Oilatum® Cream (Stiefel)

Cream, light liquid paraffin 6%, white soft paraffin 15%, net price 50 g = £1.63, 150 g = £2.46, 500-mL pump pack = £4.99, 1.05-litre pump pack = £9.98

Excipients include benzyl alcohol, cetostearyl alcohol

For dry skin conditions

Oilatum® Junior Cream (Stiefel)

Cream, light liquid paraffin 6%, white soft paraffin 15%, net price 150 g = £3.38, 350 mL = £4.65, 500 mL = £4.99, 1.05-litre pump pack = £9.98

Excipients include benzyl alcohol, cetostearyl alcohol

For dry skin conditions

QV® Cream (Sound Opinion)

Cream, glycerol 10%, light liquid paraffin 10%, white soft paraffin 5%, net price 100 g = £2.02, 500 g = £5.80, 1.05-kg pump pack = £11.80

Excipients include cetostearyl alcohol, hydroxybenzoates (parabens)

For dry skin conditions including eczema, psoriasis, ichthyosis, pruritus

QV® Intensive Ointment (Sound Opinion)

Ointment, light liquid paraffin 50.5%, white soft paraffin 20%, net price 450 g = £5.59

Excipients include cetostearyl alcohol

For dry skin conditions including eczema, psoriasis, icthyosis, pruritus

QV® Lotion (Sound Opinion)

Lotion, white soft paraffin 5%, net price 250 mL = £3.11, 500-mL pump pack = £5.18

Excipients include cetostearyl alcohol, hydroxybenzoates (parabens)

For dry skin conditions including eczema, psoriasis, ichthyosis, pruritus

Ultrabase® (Derma UK)

Cream, water-miscible, containing liquid paraffin and white soft paraffin, net price 50 g = £1.40; 500-g pump pack = £4.80

Excipients include fragrance, hydroxybenzoates (parabens), disodium edetate, stearyl alcohol

For dry skin conditions

Unguentum M® (Almirall)

Cream, saturated neutral oil, liquid paraffin, white soft paraffin, net price 50 g = £1.41, 100 g = £2.78, 200-mL pump pack = £5.50, 500 g = £8.48

Excipients include cetostearyl alcohol, polysorbate 40, propylene glycol, sorbic acid

For dry skin conditions and nappy rash

ZeroAQS® (Thornton & Ross)

Cream, macrogol cetostearyl ether 1.8%, liquid paraffin 6%, white soft paraffin 15%, net price 100 g = £1.65, 500 g = £3.29

Excipients include cetostearyl alcohol, chlorocresol

For use as an emollient or soap substitute

Zerobase® Cream (Thornton & Ross)

Cream, liquid paraffin 11%, net price 50 g = £1.04, 500-g pump pack = £5.26

Excipients include cetostearyl alcohol, chlorocresol

For dry skin conditions

Zerocream® (Thornton & Ross)

Cream, liquid paraffin 12.6%, white soft paraffin 14.5%, net price 50 g = £1.17, 500-g pump pack = £4.08

Excipients include cetyl alcohol, hydroxybenzoates (parabens), lanolin anhydrous

For dry skin conditions

Zeroguent® Cream (Thornton & Ross)

Cream, light liquid paraffin 8%, white soft paraffin 4%, refined soya bean oil 5%, net price 100 g = £2.33, 500 g = £6.99

Excipients include cetostearyl alcohol, polysorbate 40, propylene glycol, sorbic acid

For dry skin conditions

◀**Preparations containing urea, prescribe as:**

Aquadrate® (Alliance)

Cream, urea 10%, net price 100 g = £4.37

For dry, scaling and itching skin, apply thinly twice daily

Balneum® Cream (Almirall)
Cream, urea 5%, ceramide 0.1%, net price 50-g pump pack = £2.85, 500-g pump pack = £9.97
Excipients include cetostearyl alcohol, polysorbates, propylene glycol
For dry skin conditions, apply twice daily

Balneum® Plus Cream (Almirall)
Cream, urea 5%, lauromacrogols 3%, net price 100 g = £3.29, 500-g pump pack = £14.99
Excipients include benzyl alcohol, polysorbates
For dry, scaling and itching skin, apply twice daily

Dermatonics Heel Balm® (Dermatonics)
Cream, urea 25%, net price 75 mL = £3.60, 200 mL = £8.50
Excipients include beeswax, lanolin
For dry skin on soles of feet, ADULT and CHILD over 12 years, apply once daily

E45® Itch Relief Cream (Reckitt Benckiser)
Cream, urea 5%, macrogol lauryl ether 3%, net price 50 g = £2.55, 100 g = £3.47, 500-g pump pack = £14.99
Excipients include benzyl alcohol, polysorbates
For dry, scaling, and itching skin, apply twice daily

Eucerin® Intensive 10% w/w Urea Treatent Cream (Beiersdorf)
Cream, urea 10%, net price 100 mL = £7.59
Excipients include benzyl alcohol, isopropyl palmitate, wool fat
For dry skin conditions including eczema, ichthyosis, xeroderma, hyperkeratosis, apply thinly and rub into area twice daily

Eucerin® Intensive 10% w/w Urea Treatment Lotion (Beiersdorf)
Lotion, urea 10%, net price 250 mL = £7.93
Excipients include benzyl alcohol, isopropyl palmitate
For dry skin conditions including eczema, ichthyosis, xeroderma, hyperkeratosis, apply thinly and rub into area twice daily

Flexitol® Heel Balm (LaCorium)
Cream, urea 25%, net price 75 g = £3.80, 200 g = £9.40, 500 g = £14.75
Excipients include benzyl alcohol, cetostearyl alcohol, fragrance, lanolin
For dry skin on soles of feet and heels, ADULT and CHILD over 12 years, apply 1–2 times daily

Hydromol® Intensive (Alliance)
Cream, urea 10%, net price 30 g = £1.64, 100 g = £4.37
For dry, scaling and itching skin, apply thinly twice daily

Nutraplus® (Galderma)
Cream, urea 10%, net price 100 g = £4.37
Excipients include hydroxybenzoates (parabens), propylene glycol
For dry, scaling and itching skin, apply 2–3 times daily

◄Emollient bath additives and shower preparations, *prescribe as:*

Aqueous Cream
Cream, emulsifying ointment 30%, [1]phenoxyethanol 1%, in freshly boiled and cooled purified water, net price 100 g = £1.12, 500 g = £5.60
Excipients include cetostearyl alcohol
1. The BP permits use of alternative antimicrobials provided their identity and concentration are stated on the label

Aquamax® (Dermato Logical)
Wash, light liquid paraffin 8%, white soft paraffin 20%, phenoxyethanol 1%, net price 250 g = £2.99
Excipients include cetostearyl alcohol, polysorbate 60
For dry skin conditions, apply to wet or dry skin and rinse

[1]Balneum® (Almirall)
Bath oil, soya oil 84.75%, net price 200 mL = £2.48, 500 mL = £5.38, 1 litre = £10.39
Excipients include butylated hydroxytoluene, propylene glycol, fragrance
For dry skin conditions including those associated with dermatitis and eczema; add 20–60 mL/bath (INFANT 5–15 mL); do not use undiluted
1. Some pack sizes may not be prescribed on the NHS and are not listed here

Balneum Plus® Bath Oil (Almirall)
Bath oil, soya oil 82.95%, mixed lauromacrogols 15%, net price 500 mL = £6.66
Excipients include butylated hydroxytoluene, propylene glycol, fragrance
For dry skin conditions including those associated with dermatitis and eczema where pruritus also experienced; add 20 mL/bath (INFANT 5 mL) or apply to wet skin and rinse

Cetraben® Emollient Bath Additive (Genus)
Emollient bath additive, light liquid paraffin 82.8%, net price 500 mL = £5.75
For dry skin conditions, including eczema, add 1–2 capfuls/bath (CHILD 0.5–1 capful) or apply to wet skin and rinse

Dermalo® (Dermal)
Bath emollient, acetylated wool alcohols 5%, liquid paraffin 65%. Net price 500 mL = £3.44
For dermatitis, dry skin conditions including ichthyosis and pruritus of the elderly; add 15–20 mL/bath (INFANT and CHILD 5–10 mL) or apply to wet skin and rinse

Diprobath® (MSD)
Bath additive, isopropyl myristate 39%, light liquid paraffin 46%. Net price 500 mL = £6.71
For dry skin conditions including dermatitis and eczema; add 25–50 mL/bath (INFANT 10 mL); do not use undiluted

Doublebase® Emollient Bath Additive (Dermal)
Emollient bath additive, liquid paraffin 65%, net price 500 mL = £5.45
Excipients include cetostearyl alcohol
For dry skin conditions including dermatitis, ichthyosis, and pruritus of the elderly; add 15–20 mL/bath, (INFANT and CHILD 5–10 mL)

Doublebase® Emollient Shower Gel (Dermal)
Emollient Shower Gel, isopropyl myristate 15%, liquid paraffin 15%. Net price 200 g = £5.21
For dry, chapped or itchy skin conditions, apply to wet or dry skin and rinse, or apply to dry skin after showering

Doublebase® Emollient Wash Gel (Dermal)
Emollient Wash Gel, isopropyl myristate 15%, liquid paraffin 15%. Net price 200-g pump pack = £5.21
For dry, chapped, or itchy skin conditions

Hydromol® Bath and Shower Emollient (Alliance)
Bath and Shower Emollient, isopropyl myristate 13%, light liquid paraffin 37.8%. Net price 350 mL = £3.61, 500 mL = £4.11, 1 litre = £8.19
For dry skin conditions including eczema, ichthyosis and pruritus of the elderly; add 1–3 capfuls/bath (INFANT 0.5–2 capfuls) or apply to wet skin and rinse

Oilatum® Emollient (Stiefel)

Bath additive (emulsion), light liquid paraffin 63.4%. Net price 250 mL = £2.75; 500 mL = £4.57

Excipients include acetylated lanolin alcohols, isopropyl palmitate, fragrance

For dry skin conditions including dermatitis, pruritus of the elderly and ichthyosis; add 1–3 capfuls/bath (INFANT 0.5–2 capfuls) or apply to wet skin and rinse

Oilatum® Junior Bath Additive (Stiefel)

Bath additive, light liquid paraffin 63.4%, net price 150 mL = £2.82, 250 mL = £3.25, 300 mL = £5.10, 600 mL = £5.89

Excipients include acetylated lanolin alcohols, isopropyl palmitate

For dry skin conditions including dermatitis, pruritus of the elderly and ichthyosis; add 1–3 capfuls/bath (INFANT 0.5–2 capfuls) or apply to wet skin and rinse

Oilatum® Gel (Stiefel)

Shower emollient (gel), light liquid paraffin 70%, net price (with fragrance or fragrance-free) 150 g = £5.15

For dry skin conditions including dermatitis, pruritus of the elderly, and ichthyosis, apply to wet skin and rinse

QV® Bath Oil (Sound Opinion)

Bath oil, light liquid paraffin 85.13%, net price 200 mL = £2.20, 500 mL = £4.66

For dry skin conditions including eczema, psoriasis, ichthyosis, and pruritus, add 10 mL/bath (INFANT 4 mL) or apply to wet skin and rinse

QV® Gentle Wash (Sound Opinion)

Wash, glycerol 15%, net price 250 mL = £3.11, 500-mL pump pack = £5.18

Excipients include hydroxybenzoates (parabens)

For dry skin conditions including eczema, psoriasis, ichthyosis, and pruritus, use as soap substitute

Zerolatum® Emollient Medicinal Bath Oil (Thornton & Ross)

Bath Oil, liquid paraffin 65%, acetylated wool alcohols 5%, net price 500 mL = £4.79

For dry skin conditions including dermatitis, pruritus of the elderly, and ichthyosis, add 15–20 mL/bath (CHILD 5–10 mL)

Zeroneum® Bath Oil (Thornton & Ross)

Bath Oil, refined soya bean oil 83.35%, net price 500 mL = £4.48

Excipients include butylated hydroxytoluene, fragrance, propylene glycol

For dry skin conditions including eczema, add 20 mL/bath (CHILD 5 mL)

◢ DIMETICONE (SILICONE)

Dimeticone barrier creams containing at least 10%

◢ *Prescribe as:*

Dimeticone Cream (*Conotrane*)

Cream, benzalkonium chloride 0.1%, dimeticone '350' 22%. Net price 100 g = 88p; 500 g = £3.51.

Excipients include cetostearyl alcohol, fragrance

For nappy and urinary rash and pressure sores

Dimeticone Cream (*Siopel*)

Barrier cream, dimeticone '1000' 10%, cetrimide 0.3%, arachis (peanut) oil. Net price 50 g = £2.15.

Excipients include butylated hydroxytoluene, cetostearyl alcohol, hydroxybenzoates (parabens)

For protection against water-soluble irritants

◢ TITANIUM or ZINC

◢ *Prescribe as:*

Titanium Ointment

Ointment, titanium dioxide 20%, titanium peroxide 5%, titanium salicylate 3% in a basis containing dimeticone, light liquid paraffin, white soft paraffin, and benzoin tincture. Net price 30 g = £2.06. *Proprietary product: Metanium Ointment*

For nappy rash

Zinc and Castor Oil Ointment

Ointment, zinc oxide 7.5%, castor oil 50%, arachis (peanut) oil 30.5%, white beeswax 10%, cetostearyl alcohol 2%, net price 500 g = £6.00.

For nappy and urinary rash

Zinc Oxide and Dimeticone Spray

Spray application, dimeticone 1.04%, zinc oxide 12.5%, in a basis containing wool alcohols, cetostearyl alcohol, dextran, white soft paraffin, liquid paraffin, propellants. Net price 115-g pressurised aerosol unit = £8.90. *Proprietary product: Sprilon*

Excipients include cetostearyl alcohol, hydroxybenzoates (parabens), wool fat

For urinary rash, pressure sores, leg ulcers, moist eczema, fissures, fistulae and ileostomy care

Cautions flammable

Barrier preparations

Corresponds to BNF section 13.2.2.

Barrier preparations often contain water-repellent substances such as **dimeticone** (dimethicone) or other silicones. They are used on the skin around stomas, bedsores, and pressure areas in the elderly where the skin is intact. Where the skin has broken down, barrier preparations have a limited role in protecting adjacent skin. They are not a substitute for adequate nursing care. A spray preparation, **zinc oxide and dimeticone spray**, is also available.

Nappy rash The first line of treatment is to ensure that nappies are changed frequently and that tightly fitting water-proof pants are avoided. The rash may clear when left exposed to the air, and a barrier preparation, applied with each nappy change, can be helpful. If the rash is associated with candidal infection, a topical antifungal such as clotrimazole cream can be used.

Pruritus

Corresponds to BNF section 13.3.

Pruritus may be caused by systemic disease (such as obstructive jaundice, endocrine disease, chronic renal disease, iron deficiency, and certain malignant diseases), skin disease (e.g. psoriasis, eczema, urticaria, and scabies), drug hypersensitivity, or as a side-effect of opioid analgesics. Where possible, the underlying causes should be treated. An **emollient** may be of value where the pruritus is associated with dry skin (which is common in otherwise healthy elderly people).

Preparations containing **crotamiton** are sometimes used in pruritus but are of uncertain value. Crotamiton can be used to control itching after treatment with a parasiticidal preparation for scabies (see p. 20).

Preparations containing calamine are often ineffective and therefore these preparations are no longer included in the NPF.

CROTAMITON

Indications pruritus (including pruritus after scabies); see notes above

Cautions avoid use near eyes, in buccal mucosa, or on broken or very inflamed skin; use on doctor's advice for children under 3 years

Contra-indications acute exudative dermatoses

Administration pruritus, apply 2–3 times daily; CHILD under 3 years, apply once daily

◢*Prescribe as:*

Crotamiton Cream 10%
Cream, crotamiton 10%. Net price 30 g = £2.38; 100 g = £4.15. *Proprietary product: Eurax Cream*
Excipients include beeswax, fragrance, hydroxybenzoates (parabens), stearyl alcohol

Crotamiton Lotion 10%
Lotion, crotamiton 10%. Net price 100 mL = £3.14. *Proprietary product: Eurax Lotion*
Excipients include cetyl alcohol, fragrance, propylene glycol, sorbic acid, stearyl alcohol

Fungal infections

Corresponds to BNF section 13.10.2.

Fungal skin infections can be prevented by keeping the susceptible area as clean and dry as possible. Localised fungal infections such as ringworm infection and candidal skin infection can be treated with **clotrimazole cream**, **econazole cream** or **miconazole cream**.

To prevent relapse, local antifungal treatment should be continued for 1–2 weeks after the disappearance of all signs of infection. Systemic antifungal therapy is necessary for scalp infection or if the skin infection is widespread, disseminated, or intractable. There are other topical therapies (not in the Nurse Prescribers' list) to treat some nail infections but systemic treatment is more effective (see BNF Section 13.10.2).

CLOTRIMAZOLE

Indications fungal skin infections

Cautions avoid contact with eyes and mucous membranes

Pregnancy minimal absorption from skin; not known to be harmful

Side-effects occasional skin irritation or hypersensitivity reactions including mild burning sensation, erythema, and itching (discontinue if severe)

Administration apply 2–3 times daily

◢*Prescribe as:*

Clotrimazole Cream 1%
Cream, clotrimazole 1%. Net price 20 g = £1.44
Excipients are not shown because preparation available from several sources; for sensitised individuals, check that product dispensed is free from any sensitising ingredient

ECONAZOLE NITRATE

Indications see under Clotrimazole

Cautions see under Clotrimazole

Pregnancy minimal absorption from skin; not known to be harmful

Side-effects see under Clotrimazole

Administration apply twice daily

◢*Prescribe as:*

Econazole Cream 1%
Cream, econazole nitrate 1%. *Proprietary product: Pevaryl® Cream* (net price 30 g = £3.71)
Excipients include butylated hydroxyanisole, fragrance

MICONAZOLE NITRATE

Indications see under Clotrimazole

Cautions see under Clotrimazole; **interactions**: see BNF Appendix 1 (miconazole)

Pregnancy minimal absorption from skin; manufacturer advises caution

Side-effects see under Clotrimazole

Administration apply twice daily continuing for 10 days after lesions have healed

◢*Prescribe as:*

Miconazole Cream 2%
Cream, miconazole nitrate 2%. Net price 20 g = £2.05, 45 g = £1.97
Excipients are not shown because preparation available from several sources; for sensitised individuals, check that product dispensed is free from any sensitising ingredient

Boils

Boils are generally treated with a systemic antibacterial, but **magnesium sulfate paste** can be used as an adjunct when dressing the boil or carbuncle.

MAGNESIUM SULFATE

Indications paste used as an adjunct in the management of boils

Administration apply under dressing

◢*Prescribe as:*

Magnesium Sulfate Paste
Paste, dried magnesium sulfate 45 g, glycerol 55 g, phenol 500 mg. Net price 25 g = 75p, 50 g = 88p
Note Stir before use

Disinfection and cleansing

Corresponds to BNF section 13.11.

Physiological saline

Sterile **sodium chloride solution** 0.9% is suitable for general cleansing of skin and wounds but tap water is often appropriate.

 SODIUM CHLORIDE

Indications skin cleansing

◢*Prescribe as:*

Sterile Sodium Chloride Solution 0.9%
Sterile solution, sodium chloride 0.9%. To be used undiluted for topical irrigation of wounds.
Aerosol can: 100-mL can = £2.03 (*proprietary product: Stericlens*); 200-mL can = £2.65 (*proprietary product: Nine Lives*); 240-mL can = £3.09 (*proprietary products: Stericlens, Irriclens*)
Bellows Pack: 120-mL = £1.53 (*proprietary product: Flowfusor*)
Bottle: 30 × 100-mL = £19.50 (*proprietary product: MiniVersol*); 150 mL = 99p (*proprietary products include: Sterac*); 500 mL = 75p, 1 litre = 80p
Sachets and pods: 25 × 20-mL unit = £4.95 (*proprietary products include: Alissa, Clinipod, Irripod, Steripod, Sterowash*); 25 × 25-mL sachet = £6.36 (*proprietary product: Normasol*); 24 × 45-mL unit = £10.56 (*proprietary products include: MiniVersol*); 10 × 100-mL sachet = £7.73 (*proprietary product: Normasol*); other sizes also prescribable if available

Chlorhexidine

Chlorhexidine gluconate aqueous and alcoholic solutions are useful where skin disinfection is required.

 CHLORHEXIDINE

Indications skin disinfection

Cautions avoid contact with eyes, brain, meninges and middle ear; not for use in body cavities; alcoholic solutions not suitable before diathermy

Side-effects occasional sensitivity

◢*Prescribe as:*

Chlorhexidine Gluconate Alcoholic Solution
Solution, chlorhexidine gluconate solution 2.5% (≡ chlorhexidine gluconate 0.5%), in an alcoholic solution, net price 600 mL (clear) = £3.49; 600 mL (pink) = £3.49, 200-mL spray = £1.77, 500-mL spray = £3.01. *Proprietary products: Hydrex Solution, Hydrex Spray*
Note Flammable

Chlorhexidine Gluconate Alcoholic Solution
Cutaneous solution, sterile, chlorhexidine gluconate 2% in isopropyl alcohol 70%, net price (all with single applicator) 0.67 mL (with *SEPP®* applicator) = 30p, 1.5 mL (with *FREPP®* applicator) = 55p, 1.5 mL = 78p, 3 mL = 85p, 10.5 mL = £2.92, 26 mL = £6.50; (all with single applicator, with tint) 3 mL =

89p, 10.5 mL = £3.07, 26 mL = £6.83. *Proprietary product: ChloraPrep*
For skin disinfection before invasive procedures; CHILD under 2 months, not recommended
Note Flammable

Chlorhexidine Gluconate Aqueous Solution
Solution, (sterile), pink, chlorhexidine gluconate 0.05%, net price 25 × 25-mL sachet = £5.40; 10 × 100-mL sachet = £6.67. *Proprietary product: Unisept*

Povidone–iodine

Povidone–iodine aqueous solution 10% is useful where skin disinfection is required.

 POVIDONE–IODINE

Indications skin disinfection

Cautions broken skin (see below)
Large open wounds The application of povidone–iodine to large wounds or severe burns may produce systemic adverse effects such as metabolic acidosis, hypernatraemia and impairment of renal function

Contra-indications postmenstrual age under 32 weeks; avoid regular use in patients with thyroid disorders or those receiving lithium therapy

Renal impairment avoid regular application to inflamed or broken mucosa

Pregnancy sufficient iodine may be absorbed to affect the fetal thyroid in the second and third trimester

Breast-feeding avoid

Side-effects rarely sensitivity; may interfere with thyroid function tests

◢*Prescribe as:*

Povidone–Iodine Solution 10%
Solution, povidone–iodine 10% in aqueous solution. Net price 500 mL = £5.43. *Proprietary product: Videne Antiseptic Solution.*
Administration apply undiluted in pre-operative skin disinfection and general antisepsis

Wound management products and elasticated garments

See BNF Appendix 5

Wound management products and elasticated garments described as in the BNF are not in the Drug Tariff or on the Nurse Prescribers' List.

Medicated bandages and stocking

Corresponds to BNF Appendix 5.8.9.

Zinc Paste Bandage has been used with compression bandaging for the treatment of venous leg ulcers. However, paste bandages are associated with hypersensitivity reactions and should be used with caution.

Zinc paste bandages are also used with **coal tar** or **ichthammol** in chronic lichenified skin conditions such as chronic eczema (ichthammol often being preferred since its action is considered to be milder). They are also used with **calamine** in milder eczematous skin conditions.

ZINC OXIDE

Indications   see notes above

Administration   see notes above and under preparations below

◢*Prescribe as:*

Zinc Paste Bandage, BP 1993

Cotton fabric, plain weave, impregnated with suitable paste containing zinc oxide; requires additional bandaging. Net price 6 m × 7.5 cm = £3.44. *Proprietary product: Viscopaste PB7* (10%), *excipients: include* cetostearyl alcohol, hydroxybenzoates

Zinc Paste and Ichthammol Bandage, BP 1993

Cotton fabric, plain weave, impregnated with suitable paste containing zinc oxide and ichthammol; requires additional bandaging. Net price 6 m × 7.5 cm = £3.47. *Proprietary product: Ichthopaste* (6/2%), *excipients: include* cetostearyl alcohol
Uses   see BNF section 13.5

Zinc Oxide Impregnated Medicated Bandage

Cotton fabric, selvedge weave, impregnated with paste containing zinc oxide 15% (requires additional bandaging). Net price 6 m × 7.5 cm = £3.24. *Proprietary product: Steripaste*
Excipients   include polysorbate 80

Zinc Oxide Impregnated Medicated Stocking

Stocking, sterile rayon, impregnated with ointment containing zinc oxide 20%. Net price 4-pouch carton = £12.52; 10-pouch carton = £31.30. *Proprietary product: Zipzoc*
Administration   can be used under appropriate compression bandages or hosiery in chronic venous insufficiency

Peak flow meters

Corresponds to BNF section 3.1.5

When used in addition to symptom-based monitoring, peak flow monitoring has not been proven to improve asthma control in either adults or children, however measurement of peak flow may be of benefit in adult patients who are 'poor perceivers' and hence slow to detect deterioration in their asthma, and for those with more severe asthma.

Standard-range peak flow meters are suitable for both adults and children; low-range peak flow meters are appropriate for severely restricted airflow in adults and children. Patients must be given clear guidance on the action they should take if the peak flow falls below a specified level.

Peak flow charts should be issued to patients (see BNF section 3.1.5).

◢*Prescribe as:*

Standard-range peak flow meter

Conforms to standard EN ISO 23747:2007

Peak flow meter, range 60–720 litres/minute (*Proprietary product: AirZone* = £4.50); range 60–800 litres/minute (*Proprietary products include: Medi*, net price = £4.50; *MicroPeak*, £6.50; *Mini-Wright*, £6.86; *Personal Best*, £6.86; *Pocketpeak*, £6.53); range 50–800 litres/minute (*Proprietary product: Vitalograph*, £4.75, children's coloured version also available); range 60–900 litres/minute (*Proprietary product: Pinnacle* = £6.50); range 15–999 litres/minute (*Proprietary product: Piko-1*, £9.50); also replacement mouthpieces available (not interchangeable between brands)
Note   Readings from new peak flow meters are often lower than those obtained from old Wright-scale peak flow meters and the correct chart should be used

Low-range peak flow meter

Conforms to standard EN ISO 23747:2007 except for scale range

Peak flow meter, range 30–400 litres/minute, net price = £6.90 (*proprietary product: Mini-Wright*), range 40–420 litres/minute = £6.50 (*Proprietary product: Medi*), range 50–400 litres/minute = £6.53 (*proprietary product: Pocketpeak*); also replacement mouthpieces available (not interchangeable between brands)
Note   Readings from new peak flow meters are often lower than those obtained from old Wright-scale peak flow meters and the correct chart should be used

Urinary catheters and appliances

Urinary appliances

These are listed in Part IXB of the Drug Tariff (Part 5 of the Scottish Drug Tariff, Part III of the Northern Ireland Drug Tariff).

> For links to the online Drug Tariffs, see Appliances and Reagents p. 5

Urethral catheters

These are listed in Part IXA of the Drug Tariff (Part 3 of the Scottish Drug Tariff, Part III of the Northern Ireland Drug Tariff).

Maintenance of indwelling urinary catheters

Corresponds to BNF section 7.4.4.

The deposition which occurs on urinary catheters is usually chiefly composed of phosphate and to minimise this, the catheter (if latex) should be changed at least as often as every 6 weeks. If the catheter is to be left for longer periods a silicone catheter should be used together with the appropriate use of catheter maintenance solutions. Repeated blockage usually indicates that the catheter needs to be changed.

CATHETER PATENCY SOLUTIONS

Indications catheter care; see also under preparations, below

Administration to be warmed to body temperature and instilled as required, see also under preparations, below

◢*Prescribe as:*

Sodium Chloride 0.9% Catheter Maintenance Solution

Sterile solution, sodium chloride 0.9%. *Proprietary products: OptiFlo S* (Net price 50- and 100-mL sachets = £3.30), *Uriflex S* (100-mL sachet = £3.45), *Uro-Tainer Sodium Chloride* (50- and 100-mL sachets = £3.41)

For removal of clots and other debris, to be instilled as required

'Solution G' Catheter Maintenance Solution

Sterile solution, citric acid 3.23%, magnesium oxide 0.38%, sodium bicarbonate 0.7%, disodium edetate 0.01%. *Proprietary products: OptiFlo G* (Net price 50- and 100-mL sachets = £3.50), *Uriflex G* (100-mL sachet = £2.40); *Uro-Tainer Twin Suby G* (2 × 30 mL = £4.67)

For prevention of catheter encrustation and crystallisation; in very severe cases use 'Solution R'

'Solution R' Catheter Maintenance Solution

Sterile solution, citric acid 6%, gluconolactone 0.6%, magnesium carbonate 2.8%, disodium edetate 0.01%. *Proprietary products: OptiFlo R* (Net price 50- and 100-mL sachets = £3.40), *Uriflex R* (100-mL sachet = £2.40), *Uro-Tainer Twin Solutio R* (2 × 30 mL = £4.67)

For prevention of catheter encrustation and dissolution of crystallisation if 'Solution G' unsuccessful

Water

Corresponds to BNF section 9.2.2.1

◢*Prescribe as:*

Water for Injections

Net price 1-mL amp = 18p; 2-mL amp = 14p; 5-mL amp = 25p; 10-mL amp = 25p; 10-mL vial = £1.40; 20-mL amp = 92p; 50-mL amp = £1.91; 100-mL vial = £2.25

Stoma care

Corresponds to BNF section 1.8—prescribing for patients with stoma

The 3 major types of abdominal stoma are:

- colostomy
- ileostomy
- urostomy

Each requires the collection of body waste into an artificial appliance (the 'bag') attached to the body. The bags and accessories are tailored for the different types of stoma.

Colostomy In a colostomy, a stoma is formed from a cut end of colon. The output depends on the position along the colon from which the stoma is created; the further down the colon's length from which the colostomy is formed, the greater the volume of fluid that can be reabsorbed. The discharge changes from a liquid or paste-like consistency to a nearly fully formed stool mass. The nature of the discharge determines whether the bag can be drainable or non-drainable.

A *permanent colostomy* is formed by surgical removal of the diseased part of the colon. A *temporary colostomy* may be created to allow a distal part of the colon to recover from trauma (e.g. a gunshot wound, stabbing, or road traffic accident). On healing, the colon is surgically rejoined to permit normal faecal output.

Ileostomy In an ileostomy, a piece of ileum is brought to the abdominal surface following removal of varying lengths of the colon:

- pan-procto colectomy—removal of all parts of the colon
- total colectomy—removal of all of the colon apart from the rectal stump. Later, it may be possible to create an artificial pouch in the abdominal cavity which rejoins the ileum to the rectal stump, permitting normal discharge of faeces.

Urostomy A urostomy (ileal conduit) is created by the diversion of the two ureters into a piece of colon or, more commonly, ileum. The piece of intestine is brought to the abdominal surface to form a stoma. Normal gastro-intestinal function is resumed after removal of the piece to form the stoma.

Stoma appliances

The only essential prerequisites for stoma management are the collection receptacle (the 'bag') and a means of attaching it to the abdominal wall. However, practical and successful management demands, and the *Drug Tariff* permits, the supply of a range of other components.

Stoma bags and flanges   Modern stoma bags are oblong or tapered, rectangular, plastic receptacles. A circular opening is placed over the stoma. Around the opening is a flange that is used to attach the bag to the abdominal wall. A bag may be non-drainable, for use with a descending colostomy with a solid and predictable action; or it may be drainable, having a wide-necked opening with a **bag closure**, for all other types of colostomy and for an ileostomy. A bag for a urostomy has a tap for regular drainage of urine.

A bag may be one- or two-piece, depending on whether the flange is integral with the bag, or separate.

The **flange** may be attached to the abdominal wall by double-sided adhesive rings, or by the separate use of plasters or other adhesives. Skin care is important in stoma management, and a varied range of karaya-based flanges is also available. Non-adhesive flanges are available for stomas that have a solid output only.

As a colostomy stoma is much larger than that formed from ileum, a range of flange sizes is available. However, most flanges have to be cut to size by the patient, for which measuring cards are commonly provided.

A **two-piece bag** is one in which the flange is separate from the bag, and from which the bag can be detached without removing the flange from the skin. The bag is clipped to the flange, and a waist belt can be clipped to the bag. The two-piece bag permits rapid changing should the bag develop a leak.

Accessories   **Adhesive removers** are available to assist in cleaning the skin after the flange has been removed. Care must be taken to ensure that their use does not cause or aggravate skin soreness.

Bag covers of a wide range of designs and colours are available. They are particularly useful for bags that are made of transparent or semi-transparent material.

Belts are available for use with one- or two-piece bags. Their use may aid the confidence of wearers in the ability of the adhesive to keep the bag attached to the abdomen, and be necessary in wearers with irregularly shaped or distended abdomens.

Deodorants can be placed in the bag to minimise the odour from the discharge.

Filters are integral to many colostomy and ileostomy bags, and are useful for the removal of flatus from the bag. Replacement filters can be incorporated into some designs.

Irrigation/wash-out appliances are available for colostomy patients who evacuate the bowel once every 24 to 48 hours as an alternative to uncontrolled, irregular evacuation through the stoma. A cone-shaped irrigation system is inserted into the stoma, and the distal colon filled with 1–1.5 litres of warm water. Only replacement parts can be prescribed on the NHS; complete systems have to be supplied by a hospital.

Skin fillers and protectives comprise a range of aerosols, barrier creams, gels, lotions, pastes, and wipes. Fillers are used if the abdominal wall is distorted and needs levelling to allow successful attachment of the flange. Protectives are used in cases of skin soreness, but care must be taken to ensure that their use does not compromise the adhesiveness of the flange.

Stoma caps can be clipped to the flange of a two-piece bag for short periods (e.g. during swimming or sports). Their use is practicable only with colostomies that have regular faecal movements.

Tubing that may be prescribed consists of drainage tubing for urostomy bags, for use by immobile patients, or for overnight attachment to night drainage bags.

Prescribing medicines   Prescribing for patients with stoma calls for special care. The following is a brief account of some of the main points to be borne in mind.

Enemas and washouts should **not** be prescribed for patients with an ileostomy as they may cause rapid and severe dehydration.

Colostomy patients may suffer from constipation and whenever possible should be treated by increasing fluid intake or dietary fibre. **Bulk-forming drugs** (see p. 6) should be tried. If they are insufficient, as small a dose as possible of senna (see Stimulant Laxatives, p. 7) should be used.

The doctor's advice should be obtained for other complications such as diarrhoea.

New patients are usually given advice about the use of *cleansing agents, protective creams, lotions, deodorants,* or *sealants* whilst in hospital, either by the surgeon or by stoma care nurses. Voluntary organisations offer help and support to patients with stoma.

Stoma appliances and associated products

These are listed in Part IXC of the Drug Tariff (Part 6 of the Scottish Drug Tariff, Part III of the Northern Ireland Drug Tariff).

Urostomy pouches

These are listed in Part IXC of the Drug Tariff (Part 6 of the Scottish Drug Tariff, Part III of the Northern Ireland Drug Tariff).

For links to online Drug Tariffs, see Appliances and Reagents p. 5

Appliances and reagents for diabetes

Hypodermic equipment

Corresponds to BNF section 6.1.1.3.

Patients should be advised on the safe disposal of lancets, single-use syringes, and needles. Suitable arrangements for the safe disposal of contaminated waste must be made before these products are prescribed for patients who are carriers of infectious diseases.

Lancets, **needles**, **syringes**, and **accessories** are listed under Hypodermic Equipment in Part IXA of the Drug Tariff (Part III of the Northern Ireland Drug Tariff, Part 3 of the Scottish Drug Tariff).

> For links to online Drug Tariffs, see Appliances and Reagents p. 5

Monitoring agents

Corresponds to BNF section 6.1.6.

Glucose (for glucose tolerance test) is **not** on the Nurse Prescribers' List.

 ## URINALYSIS

Urine testing for glucose is useful in patients who find blood glucose monitoring difficult. Tests for glucose employ reagent strips specific to glucose.

Reagents are also available to test for ketones and protein in urine. Patients may be required to measure ketones, for example when they become unwell—see also under Blood Monitoring, below.

◀ Reagents

See BNF section 6.1.6

Reagents described as (NHS) in the BNF are not in the Drug Tariff, or on the Nurse Prescribers' List.

 ## BLOOD MONITORING

Blood **glucose** monitoring using a meter gives a direct measure of the glucose concentration at the time of the test and can detect hypoglycaemia as well as hyperglycaemia. Patients should be properly trained in the use of blood glucose monitoring systems and the appropriate action to take, based on the results obtained. Inadequate understanding of the normal fluctuations in blood glucose can lead to confusion and inappropriate action.

> **Note** In the UK blood glucose concentration is expressed in mmol/litre and Diabetes UK advises that these units should be used for self-monitoring of blood glucose. In other European countries units of mg/100 mL (or mg/dL) are commonly used.
>
> It is advisable to check that the meter is pre-set in the correct units.

If patients are required to measure **ketones**, they should be trained in the use of a ketone monitoring system and to take appropriate action on the results obtained, including when to seek medical advice. For more information on diabetic ketoacidosis, see BNF section 6.1.3.

◀ Reagents

See BNF section 6.1.6

Reagents described as (NHS) in the BNF are not in the Drug Tariff, or on the Nurse Prescribers' List.

 # Eye-drop dispensers

Eye-drop dispensers are available to aid the instillation of eye drops especially amongst the elderly, visually impaired, arthritic, or otherwise physically limited patients. Eye-drop dispensers are for use with plastic eye drop bottles, for repeat use by individual patients. Details of products available may be found in the Drug Tariff section IXA (Part 3 of the Scottish Drug Tariff, Part III of the Northern Ireland Drug Tariff).

> For links to online Drug Tariffs, see Appliances and Reagents p. 5

Fertility and gynaecological products

Vaginal pessaries (including ring and gellhorn pessaries) are listed in Part IXA of the Drug Tariff (Part 3 of the Scottish Drug Tariff, Part III of the Northern Ireland Drug Tariff).

> For links to online Drug Tariffs, see Appliances and Reagents p. 5

Contraceptive devices

Corresponds to BNF section 7.3.4

Intra-uterine devices

The intra-uterine device (IUD) is a suitable contraceptive for women of all ages irrespective of parity; however, it is less appropriate for those with an increased risk of pelvic inflammatory disease (see BNF section 7.3.4).

The healthcare professional inserting (or removing) the intra-uterine device should be fully trained in the technique and should provide full counselling backed, where available, by the patient information leaflet.

INTRA-UTERINE CONTRACEPTIVE DEVICES

Indications contraception, see BNF section 7.3.4

Cautions see BNF section 7.3.4; also anaemia, heavy menses (progestogen intra-uterine system might be preferable, BNF section 7.3.2.3), endometriosis, severe primary dysmenorrhoea, history of pelvic inflammatory disease, diabetes, fertility problems, nulliparity and young age, severely scarred uterus (including after endometrial resection) or severe cervical stenosis; drug- or disease-induced immunosuppression (risk of infection—avoid if marked immunosuppression); epilepsy (risk of seizure at time of insertion); increased risk of expulsion if inserted before uterine involution; gynaecological examination before insertion, 6–8 weeks after, then annually but counsel women to see doctor promptly in case of significant symptoms, especially pain; anticoagulant therapy (avoid if possible)

Contra-indications severe anaemia, recent sexually transmitted infection (if not fully investigated and treated), unexplained uterine bleeding, distorted or small uterine cavity, genital malignancy, active trophoblastic disease (until return to normal of urine- and plasma-gonadotrophin concentration), pelvic inflammatory disease, established or marked immunosuppression; *copper devices:* copper allergy, Wilson's disease, medical diathermy

Pregnancy remove device; if pregnancy occurs, increased likelihood that it may be ectopic

Breast-feeding not known to be harmful

Side-effects uterine or cervical perforation, displacement, expulsion; pelvic infection may be exacerbated, menorrhagia, dysmenorrhoea, allergy; *on insertion:* pain (alleviated by NSAID such as oral ibuprofen,

30 minutes before insertion) and bleeding, occasionally epileptic seizure and vasovagal attack

◢*Prescribe as:*

Ancora® 375 Ag

Intra-uterine device, copper wire with silver core, wound on vertical stem of U-shaped plastic carrier, surface area approx. 375 mm², impregnated with barium sulfate for radio-opacity, threads attached to base of vertical stem; pre-loaded in inserter, net price = £9.95

For uterine length over 6.5 cm; replacement every 5 years (see also notes in BNF section 7.3.4)

Ancora® 375 Cu

Intra-uterine device, copper wire, wound on vertical stem of U-shaped plastic carrier, surface area approx. 375 mm², impregnated with barium sulfate for radio-opacity, threads attached to base of vertical stem; pre-loaded in inserter, net price = £7.95

For uterine length over 6.5 cm; replacement every 5 years (see also notes in BNF section 7.3.4)

Copper T 380A®

Intra-uterine device, copper wire, wound on vertical stem of T-shaped plastic carrier with copper sleeve on each arm, total surface area approx. 380 mm², impregnated with barium sulfate for radio-opacity, threads attached to base of vertical stem; with loading capsule, net price = £8.95

For uterine length 6.5–9 cm; replacement every 10 years (see also notes in BNF section 7.3.4)

Flexi-T® 300

Intra-uterine device, copper wire, wound on vertical stem of T-shaped plastic carrier, surface area approx. 300 mm², impregnated with barium sulfate for radio-opacity, monofilament thread attached to base of vertical stem; preloaded in inserter, net price = £9.47

For uterine length over 5 cm; replacement every 5 years (see also notes in BNF section 7.3.4)

Flexi-T® + 380

Intra-uterine device, copper wire, wound on vertical stem of T-shaped plastic carrier with copper sleeve on each arm, total surface area approx. 380 mm² impregnated with barium sulfate for radio-opacity, monofilament thread attached to base of vertical stem; preloaded in inserter, net price = £10.06

For uterine length over 6 cm; replacement every 5 years (see also notes in BNF section 7.3.4)

GyneFix®

Intra-uterine device, 6 copper sleeves with surface area of 330 mm² on polypropylene thread, net price = £26.64

Suitable for all uterine sizes; replacement every 5 years

Load® 375

Intra-uterine device, copper wire, wound on vertical stem of U-shaped plastic carrier, surface area approx. 375 mm² impregnated with barium sulfate for radio-opacity, monofilament thread attached to base of vertical stem; preloaded in inserter, net price = £8.52

For uterine length over 7 cm; replacement every 5 years (see also notes in BNF section 7.3.4)

Mini TT 380® Slimline

Intra-uterine device, copper wire, wound on vertical stem of T-shaped plastic carrier with copper sleeves fitted flush on to distal portion of each horizontal arm, total surface area approx. 380 mm^2, impregnated with barium sulfate for radio-opacity, thread attached to base of vertical stem; easy-loading system, no capsule, net price = £12.46

For minimum uterine length 5 cm; replacement every 5 years (see also notes in BNF section 7.3.4)

Multiload® Cu375

Intra-uterine device, copper wire, surface area approx. 375 mm^2 vertical stem length 3.5 cm, net price = £9.24

For uterine length 6–9 cm; replacement every 5 years (see also notes in BNF section 7.3.4)

Multi-Safe® 375

Intra-uterine device, copper wire, wound on vertical stem of U-shaped plastic carrier, surface area approx. 375 mm^2, impregnated with barium sulfate for radio-opacity, monofilament thread attached to base of vertical stem; preloaded in inserter, net price = £8.80

For uterine length over 6–9 cm; replacement every 5 years (see also notes in BNF section 7.3.4)

Neo-Safe® T380

Intra-uterine device, copper wire, wound on vertical stem of T-shaped plastic carrier, surface area approx. 380 mm^2, impregnated with barium sulfate for radio-opacity, threads attached to base of vertical stem, net price = £13.80

For uterine length 6.5–9 cm; replacement every 5 years (see also notes in BNF section 7.3.4)

Novaplus T 380® Ag

Intra-uterine device, copper wire with silver core, wound on vertical stem of T-shaped plastic carrier, surface area approx. 380 mm^2, impregnated with barium sulfate for radio-opacity, threads attached to base of vertical stem, net price = £12.50

'Mini' size for minimum uterine length 5 cm; 'Normal' size for uterine length 6.5–9 cm; replacement every 5 years (see also notes in BNF section 7.3.4)

Novaplus T380® Cu

Intra-uterine device, copper wire, wound on vertical stem of T-shaped plastic carrier, surface area approx. 380 mm^2, impregnated with barium sulfate for radio-opacity, threads attached to base of vertical stem, net price =£10.95

'Mini' size for minimum uterine length 5 cm; 'Normal' size for uterine length 6.5–9 cm; replacement every 5 years (see also notes in BNF section 7.3.4)

Nova-T® 380

Intra-uterine device, copper wire with silver core, wound on vertical stem of T-shaped plastic carrier, surface area approx. 380 mm^2, impregnated with barium sulfate for radio-opacity, threads attached to base of vertical stem, net price = £12.97

For uterine length 6.5–9 cm; replacement every 5 years (see also notes in BNF section 7.3.4)

T-Safe® 380 Quickload

Intra-uterine device, copper wire, wound on vertical stem of T-shaped plastic carrier with copper collar on the distal portion of each arm, total surface area approx. 380 mm^2, impregnated with barium sulfate for radio-opacity, threads attached to base of vertical stem, quick-loading system, net price = £10.29

For uterine length 6.5–9 cm; replacement every 10 years (see also notes in BNF section 7.3.4)

TT 380 Slimline®

Intra-uterine device, copper wire, wound on vertical stem of T-shaped plastic carrier, with copper sleeves fitted flush on to distal portion of each horizontal arm, total surface area approx. 380 mm^2, impregnated with barium sulfate for radio-opacity, thread attached to base of vertical stem; easy-loading system, no capsule, net price = £12.46

For uterine length 6.5–9 cm; replacement every 10 years (see also notes in BNF section 7.3.4)

UT 380 Short®

Intra-uterine device, copper wire, wound on vertical stem of T-shaped plastic carrier, total surface area approx. 380 mm^2, impregnated with barium sulfate for radio-opacity, thread attached to base of vertical stem; net price = £11.22

For uterine length 5–7 cm; replacement every 5 years (see also notes in BNF section 7.3.4)

UT 380 Standard®

Intra-uterine device, copper wire, wound on vertical stem of T-shaped plastic carrier, surface area approx. 380 mm^2, impregnated with barium sulfate for radio-opacity, thread attached to base of vertical stem; net price = £11.22

For uterine length 6.5–9 cm; replacement every 5 years (see also notes in BNF section 7.3.4)

Other contraceptive devices

◀Contraceptive caps, *prescribe as:*

Soft Silicone cap

Silicone, sizes 22 mm, 26 mm, and 30 mm, net price = £15.00. *Proprietary product: FemCap*

◀Contraceptive diaphragms, *prescribe as:*

Type A Diaphragm with Flat Metal Spring

Transparent rubber with flat metal spring, sizes 55–95 mm (rising in steps of 5 mm), net price = £5.78. *Proprietary product: Reflexions*

Type B Diaphragm with coiled metal spring

Silicone with coiled metal spring, sizes 60–90 mm (rising in steps of 5 mm), net price = £8.35. *Proprietary product: Milex Omniflex*

Type C Arcing Spring Diaphragm

Silicone with arcing spring, sizes 60–90 mm (rising in steps of 5 mm), net price = £8.35. *Proprietary products: Milex Arcing Style, Ortho All-Flex*

Spermicidal contraceptives

Corresponds to BNF section 7.3.3

Spermicidal contraceptives are useful additional safeguards but do **not** give adequate protection if used alone except where fertility is already significantly diminished. They have two components: a spermicide and a vehicle which itself may have some inhibiting effect on sperm activity. Spermicidal contraceptives are suitable for use with barrier methods, such as diaphragms or caps; however they are not generally recommended for use with condoms, as there is no evidence of any additional protection compared with non-spermicidal lubricants.

Spermicidal contraceptives are not suitable for use in those with or at high risk of sexually transmitted diseases (including HIV); high frequency use of the spermicide nonoxinol '9' has been associated with genital lesions, which may increase the risk of acquiring these infections.

> Products such as petroleum jelly (*Vaseline*), baby oil and oil-based vaginal and rectal preparations are likely to damage condoms and contraceptive diaphragms made from latex rubber, and may render them less effective as a barrier method of contraception and as a protection from sexually transmitted diseases (including HIV).

Gygel®

Gel, nonoxinol '9' 2%, net price 30 g = £4.25

Excipients include hydroxybenzoates (parabens), propylene glycol, sorbic acid

Condoms no evidence of harm to latex condoms and diaphragms

Pregnancy toxicity in *animal* studies

Breast-feeding present in milk in *animal* studies

A5 Wound management products and elasticated garments

The information in this appendix corresponds to Appendix 5 of BNF 66 (September 2013). Products described as ℕℍ𝕊 in this appendix are not in the Drug Tariff, or in the Nurse Prescribers' List.

Wound dressings　　The correct dressing for wound management depends not only on the type of wound but also on the stage of the healing process. The principal stages of healing are:

- cleansing, removal of debris;
- granulation, vascularisation;
- epithelialisation.

The ideal dressing for moist wound healing needs to ensure that the wound remains:

- moist with exudate, but not macerated;
- free of clinical infection and excessive slough;
- free of toxic chemicals, particles or fibres;
- at the optimum temperature for healing;
- undisturbed by the need for frequent changes;
- at the optimum pH value.

As wound healing passes through its different stages, different types of dressings may be required to satisfy better one or other of these requirements. Under normal circumstances, a moist environment is a necessary part of the wound healing process; exudate provides a moist environment and promotes healing, but excessive exudate can cause maceration of the wound and surrounding healthy tissue. The volume and viscosity of exudate changes as the wound heals. There are certain circumstances where moist wound healing is not appropriate (e.g. gangrenous toes associated with vascular disease).

Advanced wound dressings, (section A5.2) are designed to control the environment for wound healing, for example to donate fluid (**hydrogels**), maintain hydration (**hydrocolloids**), or to absorb wound exudate (**alginates, foams**).

Practices such as the use of irritant cleansers and desloughing agents may be harmful and are largely obsolete; removal of debris and dressing remnants should need minimal irrigation with lukewarm sterile sodium chloride 0.9% solution or water.

Hydrogel, hydrocolloid, and medical grade honey dressings can be used to deslough wounds by promoting autolytic debridement; there is insufficient evidence to support any particular method of debridement for difficult-to-heal surgical wounds. Sterile larvae (maggots) are also available for biosurgical removal of wound debris.

There have been few clinical trials able to establish a clear advantage for any particular product. The choice between different dressings depends not only on the type and stage of the wound, but also on patient preference or tolerance, site of the wound, and cost. For further information, see *Buyers' Guide: Advanced wound dressings* (October 2008); NHS Purchasing and Supply Agency, Centre for Evidence-based Purchasing.

The table below gives suggestions for choices of primary dressing depending on the type of wound (a secondary dressing may be needed in some cases).

A5.1 Basic wound contact dressings

A5.1.1 Low adherence dressings

Low adherence dressings are used as interface layers under secondary absorbent dressings. Placed directly on the wound bed, non-absorbent, low adherence dressings are suitable for clean, granulating, lightly exuding wounds without necrosis, and protect the wound bed from direct contact with secondary dressings. Care must be taken to avoid granulation tissue growing into the weave of these dressings.

Tulle dressings are manufactured from cotton or viscose fibres which are impregnated with white or yellow soft paraffin to prevent the fibres from sticking, but this

Wound contact material for different types of wounds

Wound PINK (Epithelialising)		
Low Exudate	**Moderate Exudate**	
Low adherence A5.1.1 Vapour-permeable film A5.2.2 Soft polymer A.5.2.3 Hydrocolloid A5.2.4	Soft polymer A5.2.3 Foam, low absorbent A5.2.5 Alginate A5.2.6	

Wound RED (Granulating) Symptoms or signs of infection, see **Wounds with signs of infection**		
Low Exudate	**Moderate Exudate**	**Heavy Exudate**
Low adherence A5.1.1 Soft polymer A5.2.3 Hydrocolloid A5.2.4 Foam, low absorbent A5.2.5	Hydrocolloid-fibrous A5.2.4 Foam A5.2.5 Alginate A5.2.6	Foam with extra absorbency A5.2.5 Hydrocolloid-fibrous A5.2.4 Alginate A5.2.6

Wound YELLOW (Sloughy) Symptoms or signs of infection, see **Wounds with signs of infection**		
Low Exudate	**Moderate Exudate**	**Heavy Exudate**
Hydrogel A5.2.1 Hydrocolloid A5.2.4	Hydrocolloid-fibrous A5.2.4 Alginate A5.2.6	Hydrocolloid-fibrous A5.2.4 Alginate A5.2.6 Capillary-action A5.2.7

Wound BLACK (Necrotic/Eschar) Consider mechanical debridement alongside autolytic debridement		
Low Exudate or Dry	**Moderate Exudate**	**Heavy Exudate**
Hydrogel A5.2.1 Hydrocolloid A5.2.4	Hydrocolloid A5.2.4 Hydrocolloid-fibrous A5.2.4 Foam A5.2.5	Seek advice from wound care specialist

Wounds with signs of infection **Consider systemic antibacterials if appropriate;** also consider odour-absorbent dressings (section A5.2.8) For malodourous wounds with slough or necrotic tissue, consider mechanical or autolytic debridement		
Low Exudate	**Moderate Exudate**	**Heavy Exudate**
Low adherence with honey A5.3.1 Low adherence with iodine A5.3.2 Low adherence with silver A5.3.3 Hydrocolloid with silver A5.3.3 Honey—topical A5.3.1	Hydrocolloid-fibrous with silver A5.3.3 Foam with silver A5.3.3 Alginate with silver A5.3.3 Honey—topical A5.3.1 Cadexomer—iodine A5.3.2	Hydrocolloid-fibrous with silver A5.3.3 Foam, extra absorbent, with silver A5.3.3 Alginate with honey A5.3.1 Alginate with silver A5.3.3

Note In each section of this table the dressings are listed in order of increasing absorbency.
Some wound contact (primary) dressings require a secondary dressing

is only partly successful and it may be necessary to change the dressings frequently. The paraffin reduces absorbency of the dressing. Dressings with a reduced content (light loading) of soft paraffin are less liable to interfere with absorption; dressings with 'normal loading' (such as *Jelonet*®) have been used for skin graft transfer.

Knitted viscose primary dressing is an alternative to tulle dressings for exuding wounds; it can be used as the initial layer of multi-layer compression bandaging in the treatment of venous leg ulcers.

Knitted Viscose Primary Dressing, BP 1993
Warp knitted fabric manufactured from a bright viscose monofilament.
N-A Dressing®, 9.5 cm × 9.5 cm = 35p, 9.5 cm × 19 cm = 67p (Systagenix)
N-A Ultra® (silicone-coated), 9.5 cm × 9.5 cm = 33p, 9.5 cm × 19 cm = 63p (Systagenix)
Profore®, 14 cm × 20 cm = 30p (S&N Hlth.)
Tricotex®, 9.5 cm × 9.5 cm = 32p (S&N Hlth.)

Paraffin Gauze Dressing, BP 1993
(Tulle Gras). Fabric of leno weave, weft and warp threads of cotton and/or viscose yarn, impregnated with white or yellow soft paraffin, 10 cm × 10 cm, (light loading) = 25p; (normal loading) = 37p (most suppliers including Synergy Healthcare—*Paranet*® (light loading); BSN Medical—*Cuticell*® *Classic* (normal loading); S&N Hlth.—*Jelonet*® (normal loading); Neomedic—*Neotulle*® (normal loading); C D Medical—*Paragauze*® (normal loading))

Atrauman® (Hartmann)
Non-adherent knitted polyester primary dressing impregnated with neutral triglycerides, 5 cm × 5 cm = 24p, 7.5 cm × 10 cm = 26p, 10 cm × 20 cm = 59p, 20 cm × 30 cm = £1.63

A5.1.2 Absorbent dressings

Perforated film absorbent dressings are suitable only for wounds with mild to moderate amounts of exudate; they are **not** appropriate for leg ulcers or for other lesions that produce large quantities of viscous exudate. Dressings with an absorbent cellulose or polymer wadding layer are suitable for use on moderately to heavily exuding wounds.

◀ For lightly exuding wounds

Absorbent Perforated Dressing with Adhesive Border
Low-adherence primary dressing consisting of viscose and rayon absorbent pad with adhesive border.
Cosmopor E®, 5 cm × 7.2 cm = 8p, 8 cm × 10 cm = 16p, 8 cm × 15 cm = 26p, 10 cm × 20 cm = 43p, 10 cm × 25 cm = 53p, 10 cm × 35 cm = 74p (Hartmann)
Cutiplast® Steril, 5 cm × 7.2 cm = 5p, 8 cm × 10 cm = 10p, 8 cm × 15 cm = 23p, 10 cm × 20 cm = 29p, 10 cm × 25 cm = 30p, 10 cm × 30 cm = 40p (S&N Hlth.)
Leukomed®, 7.2 cm × 5 cm = 8p, 8 cm × 10 cm = 17p, 8 cm × 15 cm = 30p, 10 cm × 20 cm = 40p, 10 cm × 25 cm = 46p, 10 cm × 30 cm = 59p, 10 cm × 35 cm = 68p (BSN Medical)

Medipore® + Pad, 5 cm × 7.2 cm = 7p, 10 cm × 10 cm = 15p, 10 cm × 15 cm = 24p, 10 cm × 20 cm = 36p, 10 cm × 25 cm = 45p, 10 cm × 35 cm = 62p (3M)
Medisafe®, 6 cm × 8 cm = 8p, 8 cm × 10 cm = 13p, 8 cm × 12 cm = 23p, 9 cm × 15 cm = 29p, 9 cm × 20 cm = 34p, 9 cm × 25 cm = 36p (Neomedic)
Mepore®, 7 cm × 8 cm = 10p, 9 cm × 11 cm = 21p, 11 cm × 15 cm = 34p, 9 cm × 20 cm = 42p, 9 cm × 25 cm = 58p, 9 cm × 30 cm = 67p, 9 cm × 35 cm = 73p (Mölnlycke)
PremierPore®, 5 cm × 7 cm = 5p, 10 cm × 10 cm = 12p, 10 cm × 15 cm = 18p, 10 cm × 20 cm = 32p, 10 cm × 25 cm = 36p, 10 cm × 30 cm = 45p, 10 cm × 35 cm = 52p (Shermond)
Primapore®, 6 cm × 8.3 cm = 17p, 8 cm × 10 cm = 18p, 8 cm × 15 cm = 31p, 10 cm × 20 cm = 41p, 10 cm × 25 cm = 47p, 10 cm × 30 cm = 59p, 10 cm × 35 cm = 91p (S&N Hlth)
Softpore®, 6 cm × 7 cm = 6p, 10 cm × 10 cm = 13p, 10 cm × 15 cm = 20p, 10 cm × 20 cm = 35p, 10 cm × 25 cm = 40p, 10 cm × 30 cm = 49p, 10 cm × 35 cm = 58p (Richardson)
Sterifix®, 5 cm × 7 cm = 19p, 7 cm × 10 cm = 31p, 10 cm × 14 cm = 55p (Hartmann)
Telfa® Island, 5 cm × 10 cm = 8p, 10 cm × 12.5 cm = 27p, 10 cm × 20 cm = 35p, 10 cm × 25.5 cm = 44p, 10 cm × 35 cm = 61p (Covidien)

Absorbent Perforated Plastic Film Faced Dressing
Low-adherence primary dressing consisting of 3 layers—perforated polyester film wound contact layer, absorbent cotton pad, and hydrophobic backing. Where no size specified by the prescriber, the 5 cm size to be supplied
Askina® Pad, 10 cm × 10 cm = 20p, (B. Braun)
Cutisorb® LA, 5 cm × 5 cm = 8p, 10 cm × 10 cm = 14p, 10 cm × 20 cm = 29p (BSN Medical)
Interpose®, 5 cm × 5 cm = 9p, 10 cm × 10 cm = 15p, 10 cm × 20 cm = 32p (Frontier)
Melolin®, 5 cm × 5 cm = 16p, 10 cm × 10 cm = 26p, 20 cm × 10 cm = 51p (S&N Hlth)
Release®, 5 cm × 5 cm = 14p, 10 cm × 10 cm = 23p, 20 cm × 10 cm = 44p (Systagenix)
Skintact®, 5 cm × 5 cm = 10p, 10 cm × 10 cm = 17p, 20 cm × 10 cm = 34p (Robinson)
Solvaline N®, 5 cm × 5 cm = 9p, 10 cm × 10 cm = 17p, 10 cm × 20 cm = 34p (Activa)
Telfa®, 5 cm × 7.5 cm = 12p, 10 cm × 7.5 cm = 15p, 15 cm × 7.5 cm = 17p, 20 cm × 7.5 cm = 29p (Covidien)

◀ For moderately to heavily exuding wounds

Absorbent Cellulose Dressing with Fluid Repellent Backing
Eclypse®, 15 cm × 15 cm = 97p, 20 cm × 30 cm = £2.14, 60 cm × 40 cm = £8.15, 60 cm × 70 cm (boot-shape) = £13.78 (Advancis)
Exu-Dry®, 10 cm × 15 cm = £1.06, 15 cm × 23 cm = £2.17, 23 cm × 38 cm = £5.04 (S&N Hlth.)
Mesorb®, cellulose wadding pad with gauze wound contact layer and non-woven repellent backing, 10 cm × 10 cm = 59p, 10 cm × 15 cm = 77p, 10 cm × 20 cm = 95p, 15 cm × 20 cm = £1.36, 20 cm × 25 cm = £2.14, 20 cm × 30 cm = £2.43 (Mölnlycke)

Telfa Max®, 22.8 cm × 38 cm = £4.62, 38 cm × 45.7 cm = £5.61, 38 cm × 60.9 cm = £8.16 (Covidien)

Zetuvit® E, *non-sterile*, 10 cm × 10 cm = 6p, 10 cm × 20 cm = 8p, 20 cm × 20 cm = 14p, 20 cm × 40 cm = 26p; *sterile*, 10 cm × 10 cm = 20p, 10 cm × 20 cm = 23p, 20 cm × 20 cm = 37p, 20 cm × 40 cm = £1.04 (Hartmann)

◢ **For heavily exuding wounds**

Cutisorb® Ultra (BSN Medical)
Super absorbent cellulose and polymer primary dressing, 10 cm × 10 cm = £2.01, 20 cm × 20 cm = £6.32, 10 cm × 20 cm = £3.37, 20 cm × 30 cm = £9.53

DryMax® Extra (Aspen Medical)
Super absorbent cellulose and polymer primary dressing, 10 cm × 10 cm = £1.80, 20 cm × 20 cm = £4.20, 10 cm × 20 cm = £2.38, 20 cm × 30 cm = £4.80

KerraMax® (Crawford)
Super absorbent polyacrylate primary dressing, 10 cm × 10 cm = 91p, 10 cm × 22 cm = £1.20, 20 cm × 22 cm = £2.12, 20 cm × 30 cm = £2.43

Zetuvit® Plus (Hartmann)
Super absorbent cellulose primary dressing, 10 cm × 10 cm = 60p, 10 cm × 20 cm = 83p, 15 cm × 20 cm = 95p, 20 cm × 25 cm = £1.30, 20 cm × 40 cm = £2.00

A5.2　Advanced wound dressings

Advanced wound dressings can be used for both acute and chronic wounds. Categories for dressings in this section (A5.2) start with the least absorptive, moisture-donating hydrogel dressings, followed by increasingly more absorptive dressings. These dressings are classified according to their primary component; some dressings are comprised of several components.

A5.2.1　Hydrogel dressings

Hydrogel dressings are most commonly supplied as an amorphous, cohesive topical application that can take up the shape of a wound. A secondary, non-absorbent dressing is needed. These dressings are generally used to donate liquid to dry sloughy wounds and facilitate autolytic debridement of necrotic tissue; some also have the ability to absorb very small amounts of exudate. Hydrogel products that do not contain propylene glycol should be used if the wound is to be treated with larval therapy.

Hydrogel sheets have a fixed structure and limited fluid-handling capacity; hydrogel sheet dressings are best avoided in the presence of infection, and are unsuitable for heavily exuding wounds.

◢ **Hydrogel sheet dressings**

ActiFormCool® (Activa)
Hydrogel dressing, 5 cm × 6.5 cm = £1.70, 10 cm × 10 cm = £2.49, 20 cm × 20 cm = £7.51, 10 cm × 15 cm = £3.58

Aquaflo® (Covidien)
Hydrogel dressing, 7.5 cm diameter = £2.55, 12 cm diameter = £5.26

Gel FX® (Synergy Healthcare)
Hydrogel dressing (without adhesive border) 10 cm × 10 cm = £1.60, 15 cm × 15 cm = £3.20

Geliperm® (Geistlich)
Hydrogel sheets, 10 cm × 10 cm = £2.48

Hydrosorb® (Hartmann)
Absorbent, transparent, hydrogel sheets containing polyurethane polymers covered with a semi-permeable film, 5 cm × 7.5 cm = £1.49; 10 cm × 10 cm = £2.12; 20 cm × 20 cm = £6.37

Hydrosorb® Comfort (with adhesive border, waterproof), 4.5 cm × 6.5 cm = £1.76; 7.5 cm × 10 cm = £2.33; 12.5 cm × 12.5 cm = £3.40

Intrasite Conformable® (S&N Hlth.)
Soft non-woven dressing impregnated with *Intrasite®* gel, 10 cm × 10 cm = £1.70; 10 cm × 20 cm = £2.30; 10 cm × 40 cm = £4.10

Novogel® (Ford)
Glycerol-based hydrogel sheets, 10 cm × 10 cm = £3.07; 30 cm × 30 cm, *standard* = £13.00, *thin* = £12.27; 5 cm × 7.5 cm = £1.95; 15 cm × 20 cm = £5.86; 20 cm × 40 cm = £11.16; 7.5 cm diameter = £2.79

SanoSkin® NET (SanoMed)
Hydrogel sheet (without adhesive border), 8.5 cm × 12 cm = £2.28

Vacunet® (Protex)
Non-adherent, hydrogel coated polyester net dressing, 10 cm × 10 cm = £1.93, 10 cm × 15 cm = £2.86

◢ **Hydrogel application (amorphous)**

ActivHeal® Hydrogel (MedLogic)
Hydrogel containing guar gum and propylene glycol, 15 g = £1.39

Aquaform® (Aspen Medical)
Hydrogel containing modified starch copolymer, 8 g = £1.61, 15 g = £1.96

Askina® Gel (B. Braun)
Hydrogel containing modified starch and glycerol, 15 g = £1.92

Cutimed® (BSN Medical)
Hydrogel, 8 g = £1.58, 15 g = £1.92, 25 g = £2.83

Flexigran® (A1 Pharmaceuticals)
Hydrogel containing starch polymer and glycerol, 15 g = £1.90

GranuGel® (ConvaTec)
Hydrogel containing carboxymethylcellulose, pectin, and propylene glycol, 15 g = £2.19

Intrasite® Gel (S&N Hlth.)
Hydrogel containing modified carmellose polymer and propylene glycol, 8-g sachet = £1.70, 15-g sachet = £2.28, 25-g sachet = £3.38

Nu-Gel® (Systagenix)
Hydrogel containing alginate and propylene glycol, 15 g = £2.09

Purilon® Gel (Coloplast)
Hydrogel containing carboxymethylcellulose and calcium alginate, 8 g = £1.64, 15 g = £2.14

A5.2.1.1 Sodium hyaluronate dressings

The hydrating properties of sodium hyaluronate promote wound healing, and dressings can be applied directly to the wound, or to a primary dressing (a secondary dressing should also be applied). The iodine and potassium iodide in these dressings prevent the bacterial decay of sodium hyaluronate in the wound.

Hyiodine® (H&R)
Sodium hyaluronate 1.5%, potassium iodide 0.15%, iodine 0.1%, in a viscous solution, 22-g = £19.95, 50-g = £35.00
Cautions thyroid disorders

A5.2.2 Vapour-permeable films and membranes

Vapour-permeable films and membranes allow the passage of water vapour and oxygen but are impermeable to water and micro-organisms, and are suitable for lightly exuding wounds. They are highly conformable, provide protection, and a moist healing environment; transparent film dressings permit constant observation of the wound. Water vapour loss can occur at a slower rate than exudate is generated, so that fluid accumulates under the dressing, which can lead to tissue maceration and to wrinkling at the adhesive contact site (with risk of bacterial entry). Newer versions of these dressings have increased moisture vapour permeability. Despite these advances, vapour-permeable films and membranes are unsuitable for infected, large heavily exuding wounds, and chronic leg ulcers.

Vapour-permeable films and membranes are suitable for partial-thickness wounds with minimal exudate, or wounds with eschar. Most commonly, they are used as a secondary dressing over alginates or hydrogels; film dressings can also be used to protect the fragile skin of patients at risk of developing minor skin damage caused by friction or pressure.

◢Vapour-permeable Adhesive Film Dressing (Semi-permeable Adhesive Dressing)
Extensible, waterproof, water vapour-permeable polyurethane film coated with synthetic adhesive mass; transparent. Supplied in single-use pieces.

ActivHeal® Film (MedLogic)
Film dressing, 6 cm × 7 cm = 32p, 10 cm × 12.7 cm = 74p, 15 cm × 17.8 cm = £1.81

Askina® Derm (B.Braun)
Film dressing, 6 cm × 7 cm = 36p, 10 cm × 12 cm = £1.04, 10 cm × 20 cm = £1.97, 15 cm × 20 cm = £2.39, 20 cm × 30 cm = £4.27

Bioclusive® (Systagenix)
Film dressing, 10.2 cm × 12.7 cm = £1.54

C-View® (Aspen Medical)
Film dressing, 6 cm × 7 cm = 38p, 10 cm × 12 cm = £1.02, 12 cm × 12 cm = £1.09, 15 cm × 20 cm = £2.36

Hydrofilm® (Hartmann)
Film dressing, 6 cm × 7 cm = 21p, 10 cm × 12.5 cm = 40p, 10 cm × 15 cm = 50p, 10 cm × 25 cm = 77p, 12 cm × 25 cm = 81p, 15 cm × 20 cm = 92p, 20 cm × 30 cm = £1.52

Hypafix® Transparent (BSN Medical)
Film dressing, 10 cm × 2 m = £8.24

Leukomed T® (BSN Medical)
Film dressing, 7.2 cm × 5 cm = 35p, 8 cm × 10 cm = 66p, 10 cm × 12.5 cm = 96p, 11 cm × 14 cm = £1.16, 15 cm × 20 cm = £2.23, 15 cm × 25 cm = £2.38

Mepore® Film (Mölnlycke)
Film dressing, 6 cm × 7 cm = 44p, 10 cm × 12 cm = £1.18, 10 cm × 25 cm = £2.29, 15 cm × 20 cm = £2.91

OpSite® Flexifix (S&N Hlth.)
Film dressing, 5 cm × 1 m = £3.69, 10 cm × 1 m = £6.22; *OpSite® Flexigrid*, 6 cm × 7 cm = 37p, 12 cm × 12 cm = £1.06, 15 cm × 20 cm = £2.69

Polyskin® II (Covidien)
Film dressing, 4 cm × 4 cm = 36p, 5 cm × 7 cm = 39p, 10 cm × 12 cm = £1.01, 10 cm × 20 cm = £2.00, 15 cm × 20 cm = £2.31, 20 cm × 25 cm = £4.03

ProtectFilm® (Wallace Cameron)
Film dressing, 6 cm × 7 cm = 11p, 10 cm × 12 cm = 20p, 15 cm × 20 cm = 40p

Suprasorb F® (Activa)
Film dressing, 5 cm × 7 cm = 32p, 10 cm × 12 cm = 76p, 15 cm × 20 cm = £2.37

Tegaderm® (3M)
Film dressing, 6 cm × 7 cm = 38p, 12 cm × 12 cm = £1.09, 15 cm × 20 cm = £2.37
Tegaderm® diamond, film dressing, 6 cm × 7 cm = £0.44, 10 cm × 12 cm = £1.19

Vacuskin® (Protex)
Film dressing, 6 cm × 7 cm = 40p, 10 cm × 12 cm = £1.06, 10 cm × 25 cm = £2.06, 15 cm × 20 cm = £2.19

Vellafilm® (Advancis)
Film dressing, 12 cm × 12 cm = £1.10, 12 cm × 35 cm = £2.75, 15 cm × 20 cm = £2.10

◢Vapour-permeable Adhesive Film Dressing with absorbent pad

Alldress® (Mölnlycke)
Film dressing, with absorbent pad, 10 cm × 10 cm = 91p, 15 cm × 15 cm = £1.98, 15 cm × 20 cm = £2.44

Clearpore® (Richardson)
Film dressing, with absorbent pad, 6 cm × 7 cm = 12p, 6 cm × 10 cm = 15p, 10 cm × 10 cm = 20p, 10 cm × 30 cm = 65p, 15 cm × 10 cm = 24p, 20 cm × 10 cm = 36p, 25 cm × 10 cm = 40p

C-View® Post-Op (Aspen Medical)
Film dressing, with absorbent pad, 6 cm × 7 cm = £0.40, 10 cm × 12 cm = £1.10, 10 cm × 25 cm = £1.60, 10 cm × 35 cm = £2.60

Hydrofilm® Plus (Hartmann)
Film dressing, with absorbent pad, 5 cm × 7.2 cm =
15p, 9 cm × 10 cm = 20p, 9 cm × 15 cm = 22p,
10 cm × 20 cm = 35p, 10 cm × 25 cm = 37p,
10 cm × 30 cm = 54p

Leukomed T® Plus (BSN Medical)
Film dressing, with absorbent pad, 7.2 cm x 5 cm =
25p, 8 cm x 10 cm = 51p, 8 cm x 15 cm = 76p,
10 cm x 20 cm = £1.26, 10 cm x 25 cm = £1.42,
10 cm x 30 cm = £2.38, 10 cm x 35 cm = £2.88

Mepore® (Mölnlycke)
Mepore® Film & Pad, film dressing, with absorbent
pad, 4 cm × 5 cm = 23p, 5 cm × 7 cm = 24p, 9 cm
× 10 cm = 61p, 9 cm × 15 cm = 90p, 9 cm ×
20 cm = £1.31, 9 cm × 25 cm = £1.47, 9 cm ×
30 cm = £1.97, 9 cm × 35 cm = £2.45

Mepore® Ultra, film dressing, with absorbent pad,
6 cm × 7 cm = 28p, 7 cm × 8 cm = 39p, 9 cm ×
10 cm = 61p, 9 cm × 15 cm = 92p, 9 cm × 20 cm
= £1.43, 9 cm × 25 cm = £1.58, 9 cm × 30 cm =
£2.61, 10 cm × 11 cm = 75p, 11 cm × 15 cm =
£1.12

OpSite® (S&N Hlth.)
OpSite® Plus, film dressing, with absorbent pad,
6.5 cm × 5 cm = 30p, 9.5 cm × 8.5 cm = 83p,
10 cm × 12 cm = £1.13, 10 cm × 20 cm = £1.90,
35 cm × 10 cm = £3.15

OpSite® Post-op, film dressing, with absorbent pad,
8.5 cm × 9.5 cm = 82p, 8.5 cm × 15.5 cm = £1.13,
10 cm × 12 cm = £1.11, 10 cm × 20 cm = £1.86,
10 cm × 25 cm = £2.35, 10 cm × 30 cm = £2.78,
10 cm × 35 cm = £3.09

Pharmapore-PU® (Wallace Cameron)
Film dressing, with absorbent pad, 8.5 cm ×
15.5 cm = 20p, 10 cm × 25 cm = 38p, 10 cm ×
30 cm = 58p

PremierPore VP® (Shermond)
Film dressing, with absorbent pad, 5 cm × 7 cm =
13p, 6 cm × 7 cm = 21p, 10 cm × 10 cm = 16p,
10 cm × 15 cm = 24p, 10 cm × 20 cm = 36p,
10 cm × 25 cm = 38p, 10 cm × 30 cm = 57p,
10 cm × 35 cm = 69p

Tegaderm® (3M)
Film dressing, with absorbent pad, 5 cm × 7 cm =
25p, 9 cm × 10 cm = 63p, 9 cm × 15 cm = 93p,
9 cm × 20 cm = £1.36, 9 cm × 25 cm = £1.53, 9 cm
× 35 cm = £2.53

Tegaderm® Absorbent Clear, film dressing, with
clear acrylic polymer oval-shaped pad, 7.6 cm ×
9.5 cm = £3.02, 11.1 cm × 12.7 cm = £3.91, 14.2 cm
× 15.8 cm = £5.51; rectangular pad, 14.9 cm ×
15.2 cm = £8.26, 20 cm × 20.3 cm = £13.26;
16.8 cm × 19 cm (sacral) = £9.89

◀ **For intravenous and subcutaneous catheter sites**

Central Gard® (Unomedical)
Vapour–permeable transparent film dressing with
adhesive foam border, 16 cm × 7 cm (central
venous catheter) = 94p, 16 cm × 8.8 cm (central
venous catheter) = £1.03

EasI-V® (ConvaTec)
Vapour–permeable transparent film dressing with
adhesive foam border, 7 cm × 7.5 cm (intravenous
peripheral cannula) = 38p

Hydrofilm® I.V. Control (Hartmann)
Vapour-permeable, transparent, adhesive film
dressing, 7 cm x 9 cm = 29p

IV3000® (S&N Hlth.)
Vapour–permeable, transparent, adhesive film
dressing, 5 cm × 6 cm (1-hand) = 40p, 6 cm ×
7 cm (non-winged peripheral catheter) = 52p, 7 cm
× 9 cm (ported peripheral catheter) = 69p, 9 cm ×
12 cm (PICC line) = £1.37, 10 cm × 12 cm (central
venous catheter) = £1.32

Mepore® IV (Mölnlycke)
Vapour–permeable, transparent, adhesive film
dressing, 5 cm × 5.5 cm = 29p, 8 cm × 9 cm =
38p, 10 cm × 11 cm = 99p

Niko Fix® (Unomedical)
Non-woven fabric dressing with viscose-rayon pad,
7 cm × 8.5 cm (intravenous ported peripheral
catheter) = 19p

Pharmapore-PU® IV (Wallace Cameron)
Vapour–permeable, transparent, adhesive film
dressing, 8.5 cm × 7 cm = 7p, 6 cm × 7 cm (ported
peripheral cannula) = 8p, 7 cm × 9 cm (peripheral
cannula, hand) = 17p

Tegaderm® IV (3M)
Vapour–permeable, transparent, adhesive film
dressing, 7 cm × 8.5 cm (peripheral catheter) = 58p,
8.5 cm × 10.5 cm (central venous catheter) = £1.12,
10 cm × 15.5 cm (peripherally inserted central
venous catheter) = £1.62

A5.2.3   Soft polymer dressings

Dressings with soft polymer, often a soft silicone polymer, in a non-adherent or gently adherent layer are
suitable for use on lightly to moderately exuding
wounds. For moderately to heavily exuding wounds,
an absorbent secondary dressing can be added, or a soft
polymer dressing with an absorbent pad can be used.

Wound contact dressings coated with soft silicone have
gentle adhesive properties and can be used on fragile
skin areas or where it is beneficial to reduce the frequency of primary dressing changes.

Soft polymer dressings should not be used on heavily
bleeding wounds; blood clots can cause the dressing to
adhere to the wound surface.

For *silicone keloid dressings* see section A5.4.2.

◀ **Without absorbent pad**

Adaptic® Touch (Systagenix)
Non-adherent soft silicone wound contact dressing,
5 cm x 7.6 cm = £1.13, 7.6 cm x 11 cm = £2.25,
12.7 cm x 15 cm = £4.65, 20 cm x 32 cm = £12.50

Askina® SilNet (B. Braun)
Soft silicone-coated wound contact dressing, 5 cm x
7.5 cm = £1.09, 7.5 cm x 10 cm = £2.20, 10 cm x
18 cm = £4.80, 20 cm x 30 cm = £11.75

Mepitel® (Mölnlycke)
Soft silicone, semi-transparent wound contact
dressing, 5 cm × 7 cm = £1.57, 8 cm × 10 cm =
£3.13, 12 cm × 15 cm = £6.34, 20 cm × 30 cm =
£16.61

Mepitel® One, soft silicone, thin, transparent wound contact dressing, 6 cm × 7 cm = £1.79, 9 cm × 10 cm = £3.36, 13 cm × 15 cm = £6.54, 24 cm × 27.5 cm = £16.79

Physiotulle® (Coloplast)
Non-adherent soft polymer wound contact dressing, 10 cm × 10 cm = £2.13, 15 cm × 20 cm = £6.50

Silon-TSR® (Jobskin)
Soft silicone polymer wound contact dressing, 13 cm × 13 cm = £3.52, 13 cm × 25 cm = £5.47, 28 cm × 30 cm = £7.37

Silflex® (Advancis)
Soft silicone-coated polyester wound contact dressing, 5 cm × 7 cm = £1.25, 8 cm × 10 cm = £2.55, 12 cm × 15 cm = £5.15, 20 cm × 30 cm = £13.25, 35 cm × 60 cm = £39.54

Sorbion® Contact (H&R)
Non-adherent soft polymer wound contact dressing, 7.5 cm × 7.5 cm = £1.49, 10 cm × 10 cm = £1.99, 10 cm × 20 cm = £3.99, 20 cm × 20 cm = £6.99, 20 cm × 30 cm = £9.99

Tegaderm® Contact (3M)
Non-adherent soft polymer wound contact dressing, 7.5 cm × 10 cm = £2.17, 7.5 cm × 20 cm = £4.25, 20 cm × 25 cm = £10.35

Urgotul® (Urgo)
Non-adherent soft polymer wound contact dressing, 5 cm × 5cm = £1.50, 10 cm × 10 cm = £3.00, 10 cm × 40 cm = £10.08, 15 cm × 15 cm = £6.45, 15 cm × 20 cm = £8.49, 20 cm × 30 cm = £13.65

◢ With absorbent pad

Advazorb® Silfix (Advancis)
Soft silicone wound contact dressing, with polyurethane foam film backing, 7.5 cm × 7.5 cm = £0.99, 10 cm × 10 cm = £1.85, 10 cm × 20 cm = £3.18, 12.5 cm × 12.5 cm = £2.59, 15 cm × 15 cm = £3.36, 20 cm × 20 cm = £4.98

Advazorb® Silfix Lite, soft silicone wound contact dressing, with polyurethane foam film backing, 7.5 cm × 7.5 cm = £0.89, 10 cm × 10 cm = £1.67, 10 cm × 20 cm = £2.86, 12.5 cm × 12.5 cm = £2.33, 15 cm × 15 cm = £3.02, 20 cm × 20 cm = £4.48

Advazorb® Silflo (Advancis)
Soft silicone wound contact dressing, with polyurethane foam film backing and adhesive border, 7.5 cm × 7.5 cm = £1.19, 10 cm × 10 cm = £2.10, 10 cm × 20 cm = £2.90, 10 cm × 30 cm = £4.25, 12.5 cm × 12.5 cm = £2.58, 15 cm × 15 cm = £3.15, 20 cm × 20 cm = £5.46

Advazorb® Silflo Lite, soft silicone wound contact dressing, with polyurethane foam film backing and adhesive border, 7.5 cm × 7.5 cm = £1.07, 10 cm × 10 cm = £1.89, 10 cm × 20 cm = £2.61, 10 cm × 30 cm = £3.83, 12.5 cm × 12.5 cm = £2.32, 15 cm × 15 cm = £2.84, 20 cm × 20 cm = £4.91

Allevyn® Gentle (S&N Hlth.)
Soft gel wound contact dressing, with polyurethane foam film backing, 5 cm × 5 cm = £1.21, 10 cm × 10 cm = £2.40, 10 cm × 20 cm = £3.86, 15 cm × 15 cm = £4.03, 20 cm × 20 cm = £6.44

Allevyn® Gentle Border, silicone gel wound contact dressing, with polyurethane foam film backing, 7.5 cm × 7.5 cm = £1.43, 10 cm × 10 cm = £2.10, 12.5 cm × 12.5 cm = £2.57, 17.5 cm × 17.5 cm = £5.07, 23 cm × 23.2 cm (heel) = £9.24

Allevyn® Gentle Border Lite, silicone gel wound contact dressing, with polyurethane foam film backing, 5 cm x 5 cm = 86p, 5.5 cm x 12 cm = £1.77, 7.5 cm x 7.5 cm = £1.33, 8 cm x 15 cm = £3.29, 10 cm x 10 cm = £2.07, 15 cm x 15 cm = £3.65

Allevyn® Life (S&N Hlth)
Soft silicone wound contact dressing, with central mesh screen, polyurethane foam film backing and adhesive border, 10.3 cm × 10.3 cm = £1.65, 12.9 cm × 12.9 cm = £2.42, 15.4 cm × 15.4 cm = £2.96, 21 cm × 21 cm = £5.83

Cutimed® Siltec (BSN Medical)
Soft silicone wound contact dressing, with polyurethane foam film backing, 5 cm × 6 cm = £1.24, 10 cm × 10 cm = £2.33, 10 cm × 20 cm = £3.84, 15 cm × 15 cm = £4.35, 20 cm × 20 cm = £6.59, 16 cm × 24 cm (heel) = £6.77; with adhesive border, 17.5 cm × 17.5 cm (sacrum) = £4.31, 23 cm x 23 cm (sacrum) = £7.02

Cutimed® Siltec B, with adhesive border, for lightly to moderately exuding wounds, 7.5 cm × 7.5 cm = £1.45, 12.5 cm × 12.5 cm = £3.06, 15 cm × 15 cm = £4.71, 17.5 cm × 17.5 cm = £4.97, 22.5 cm x 22.5 cm = £8.16

Cutimed® Siltec L, for lightly to moderately exuding wounds, 5 cm × 6 cm = 99p, 10 cm × 10 cm = £2.00, 15 cm × 15 cm = £3.30

Eclypse® Adherent (Advancis)
Soft silicone wound contact layer with absorbent pad and film-backing, 10 cm × 10 cm = £2.99, 10 cm × 20 cm = £3.75, 15 cm × 15 cm = £4.99, 20 cm × 30 cm = £9.99, 17 cm × 19 cm (sacral) = £3.76, 22 cm × 23 cm (sacral) = £6.23

Flivasorb® (Activa)
Absorbent polymer dressing with non-adherent wound contact layer, 10 cm × 10 cm = £2.16, 20 cm × 20 cm = £6.80, 10 cm × 20 cm = £3.61, 20 cm × 30 cm = £9.62

Flivasorb® Adhesive, absorbent polymer dressing with non-adherent wound contact layer and adhesive border, 12 cm × 12 cm = £3.25, 15 cm × 15 cm = £4.45

Mepilex® (Mölnlycke)
Absorbent soft silicone dressing with polyurethane foam film backing, 10 cm × 11 cm = £2.57, 11 cm × 20 cm = £4.24, 15 cm × 16 cm = £4.66, 20 cm × 21 cm = £7.03, 20 cm × 50 cm = £27.76, 13 cm × 20 cm (heel) = £5.22, 15 cm × 22 cm (heel) = £6.01

Mepilex® Border, absorbent soft silicone dressing with polyurethane foam and adhesive border, 7 cm × 7.5 cm = £1.33, 10 cm × 12.5 cm = £2.63, 10 cm × 20 cm = £3.56, 10 cm × 30 cm = £5.36, 15 cm × 17.5 cm = £4.53, 17 cm × 20 cm = £5.87, 18 cm × 18 cm (sacrum) = £4.69, 23 cm × 23 cm (sacrum) = £7.64

Mepilex® Border Lite, thin absorbent soft silicone dressing with polyurethane foam and adhesive border, 4 cm × 5 cm = 91p, 7.5 cm × 7.5 cm = £1.37, 5 cm × 12.5 cm = £1.98, 10 cm × 10 cm = £2.49, 15 cm × 15 cm = £4.06

Mepilex® Lite, thin absorbent soft silicone dressing with polyurethane foam, 6 cm × 8.5 cm = £1.74, 10 cm × 10 cm = £2.08, 15 cm × 15 cm = £4.03, 20 cm × 50 cm = £25.46

Mepilex® Transfer, soft silicone exudate transfer dressing, 7.5 cm × 8.5 cm = £2.13, 10 cm × 12 cm = £3.35, 15 cm × 20 cm = £10.16, 20 cm × 50 cm = £25.97

Sorbion® Sana (H&R)
Non-adherent polyethylene wound contact dressing with absorbent core, 8.5 cm × 8.5 cm = £5.00, 12 cm × 12 cm = £6.78, 12 cm × 22 cm = £12.56, 22 cm × 22 cm = £20.14

Urgotul® Duo (Urgo)
Non-adherent, soft polymer wound contact dressing with absorbent pad, 5 cm × 10 cm = £2.33, 10 cm × 12 cm = £3.61, 15 cm × 20 cm = £8.38
Urgotul® Duo Border, soft polymer wound contact dressing with absorbent pad and adhesive polyurethane film backing, 8 cm × 8 cm = £2.27, 10 cm × 12 cm = £3.52, 15 cm × 20 cm = £8.17

◢Cellulose dressings

Sorbion® Sachet (H&R)
Sorbion® Sachet Border, absorbent polymers in cellulose matrix, hypoallergenic polypropylene envelope, with adhesive border (for moderately to heavily exuding wounds), 10 cm × 10 cm = £2.95, 15 cm × 15 cm = £4.49, 15 cm × 25 cm = £6.99, 25 cm × 25 cm = £11.99
Sorbion® Sachet Drainage, absorbent polymers in cellulose matrix, hypoallergenic polypropylene envelope ('v' shaped dressing), 10 cm × 10 cm = £2.64
Sorbion® Sachet EXTRA, absorbent polymers in cellulose matrix, hypoallergenic polypropylene envelope (for moderately to heavily exuding wounds), 5 cm × 5 cm =£1.45, 7.5 cm × 7.5 cm = £1.78, 10 cm × 10 cm = £2.25, 10 cm × 20 cm = £3.73, 20 cm × 20 cm = £7.00, 30 cm × 20 cm = £9.99
Sorbion® Sachet Multi Star, absorbent polymers in cellulose matrix, hypoallergenic polypropylene envelope (for moderately to heavily exuding wounds), 8 cm × 8 cm = £2.99, 14 cm × 14 cm = £4.89

Suprasorb® X (Activa)
Biosynthetic cellulose fibre dressing (for lightly to moderately exuding wounds), 5 cm × 5 cm = £1.93, 9 cm × 9 cm = £4.02, 14 cm × 20 cm = £7.96; 2 cm × 21 cm (rope) = £6.19

A5.2.4 Hydrocolloid dressings

Hydrocolloid dressings are usually presented as a hydrocolloid layer on a vapour-permeable film or foam pad. Semi-permeable to water vapour and oxygen, these dressings form a gel in the presence of exudate to facilitate rehydration in lightly to moderately exuding wounds and promote autolytic debridement of dry,

sloughy, or necrotic wounds; they are also suitable for promoting granulation.

Hydrocolloid-fibrous dressings made from modified carmellose fibres resemble alginate dressings; hydro-colloid-fibrous dressings are more absorptive and suitable for moderately to heavily exuding wounds.

◢Without adhesive border

ActivHeal® Hydrocolloid (MedLogic)
Semi-permeable polyurethane film backing, hydrocolloid wound contact layer, 5 cm × 7.5 cm = 76p, 10 cm × 10 cm = £1.55, 15 cm × 15 cm = £3.37, 15 cm × 18 cm (sacral) = £3.91; *with polyurethane foam layer*, 5 cm × 7.5 cm = 96p, 10 cm × 10 cm = £1.52, 15 cm × 15 cm = £2.86, 15 cm × 18 cm (sacral) = £3.30

Askina® Biofilm Transparent (B. Braun)
Semi-permeable, polyurethane film dressing with hydrocolloid adhesive, 10 cm × 10 cm = £1.02, 20 cm × 20 cm = £3.02

Biatain® Super (Coloplast)
Semi–permeable hydrocolloid dressing without adhesive border, 10 cm × 10 cm = £3.12, 12.5 cm × 12.5 cm = £4.29, 12 cm × 20 cm = £5.63, 15 cm × 15 cm = £5.43, 20 cm × 20 cm = £8.10

Comfeel® Plus (Coloplast)
Hydrocolloid dressings containing carmellose sodium and calcium alginate. *contour*, 6 cm × 8 cm = £2.08, 9 cm × 11 cm = £3.61; *ulcer*, 4 cm × 6 cm = 90p, 10 cm × 10 cm = £2.29, 15 cm × 15 cm = £4.91, 18 cm × 20 cm (triangular) = £5.35, 20 cm × 20 cm = £7.08; *transparent*, 5 cm × 7 cm = 63p, 5 cm × 15 cm = £1.48, 5 cm × 25 cm = £2.41, 9 cm × 14 cm = £2.28, 9 cm × 25 cm = £3.24, 10 cm × 10 cm = £1.20, 15 cm × 15 cm = £3.12, 15 cm × 20 cm = £3.17, 20 cm × 20 cm = £3.19; *pressure relieving*, 7 cm diameter = £3.24, 10 cm diameter = £4.34, 15 cm diameter = £6.54

DuoDERM® Extra Thin (ConvaTec)
Semi-permeable hydrocolloid dressing, 5 cm × 10 cm = 72p, 7.5 cm × 7.5 cm = 75p, 10 cm × 10 cm = £1.24, 9 cm × 15 cm = £1.66, 9 cm × 25 cm = £2.66, 9 cm × 35 cm = £3.72, 15 cm × 15 cm = £2.68

DuoDERM® Signal, **hydrocolloid dressing with** 'Time to change' indicator, 10 cm × 10 cm = £2.00, 14 cm × 14 cm = £3.52, 20 cm × 20 cm = £6.99, 11 cm × 19 cm (oval) = £3.05, 18.5 cm × 19.5 cm (heel) = £4.92, 22.5 cm × 20 cm (sacral) = £5.74

Flexigran® (A1 Pharmaceuticals)
Semi-permeable hydrocolloid dressing without adhesive border, 10 cm × 10 cm = £2.19; *thin*, 10 cm × 10 cm = £1.08

Granuflex® (ConvaTec)
Hydrocolloid wound contact layer bonded to plastic foam layer, with outer semi-permeable polyurethane film, 10 cm × 10 cm = £2.64, 15 cm × 15 cm = £5.00, 15 cm × 20 cm = £5.42, 20 cm × 20 cm = £7.52

Hydrocoll® Basic (Hartmann)
Hydrocolloid dressing with absorbent wound contact pad, 10 cm × 10 cm = £2.32; *thin*, 7.5 cm × 7.5 cm = 66p, 10 cm × 10 cm = £1.09, 15 cm × 15 cm = £2.46

NU DERM® (Systagenix)

Semi-permeable hydrocolloid dressing, 5 cm × 5 cm = 85p, 10 cm × 10 cm = £1.56, 15 cm × 15 cm = £3.18, 20 cm × 20 cm = £6.36, 8 cm × 12 cm (heel/elbow) = £3.18, 15 cm × 18 cm (sacral) = £4.45; *thin*, 10 cm × 10 cm = £1.06

Tegaderm® **Hydrocolloid** (3M)

Hydrocolloid dressing without adhesive border, 10 cm × 10 cm = £2.30, 15 cm × 15 cm = £4.46; *thin*, semi-permeable, clear film dressing with hydrocolloid, 10 cm × 10 cm = £1.51

Ultec Pro® (Covidien)

Semi-permeable hydrocolloid dressing; without adhesive border 10 cm × 10 cm = £2.23, 15 cm × 15 cm = £4.36, 20 cm × 20 cm = £6.56

◢With adhesive border

Biatain® **Super** (Coloplast)

Semi-permeable hydrocolloid dressing with adhesive border, 10 cm × 10 cm = £3.12, 12.5 cm × 12.5 cm = £4.29, 12 cm × 20 cm = £5.63, 15 cm × 15 cm = £5.43, 20 cm × 20 cm = £8.10

Granuflex® **Bordered** (ConvaTec)

Hydrocolloid wound contact layer bonded to plastic foam layer, with outer semi-permeable polyurethane film, 6 cm × 6 cm = £1.66, 10 cm × 10 cm = £3.14, 15 cm × 15 cm = £5.99, 10 cm × 13 cm (triangular) = £3.71, 15 cm × 18 cm (triangular) = £5.78

Hydrocoll® **Border** (Hartmann)

Hydrocolloid dressing with adhesive border and absorbent wound contact pad, 5 cm × 5 cm = 95p, 7.5 cm × 7.5 cm = £1.57, 10 cm × 10 cm = £2.29, 15 cm × 15 cm = £4.30; 8 cm × 12 cm (concave) = £2.01; 12 cm × 18 cm (sacral) = £3.42

Tegaderm® **Hydrocolloid** (3M)

Hydrocolloid dressing with adhesive border, 10 cm × 12 cm (oval) = £2.26, 13 cm × 15 cm (oval) = £4.22; 17.1 cm × 16.1 cm (sacral) = £4.71; *thin*, semi-permeable, clear film dressing with hydrocolloid, 10 cm × 12 cm (oval) = £1.50; 13 cm × 15 cm (oval) = £2.81

Ultec Pro® (Covidien)

Semi-permeable hydrocolloid dressing with adhesive border, 21 cm × 21 cm = £4.58, 15 cm × 18 cm (sacral) = £3.23, 19.5 cm × 23 cm (sacral) = £4.88

◢Hydrocolloid-fibrous dressings

Aquacel® (ConvaTec)

Soft non-woven pad containing hydrocolloid-fibres, 4 cm × 10 cm = £1.40, 4 cm × 20 cm = £2.07, 4 cm × 30 cm = £3.11, 5 cm × 5 cm = £1.10; 10 cm × 10 cm = £2.61; 15 cm × 15 cm = £4.91; 1 cm × 45 cm (ribbon) = £1.76, 2 cm × 45 cm (ribbon) = £2.64

Aquacel® Foam, soft non-woven pad containing hydrocolloid-fibres with foam layer, without adhesive border, 5 cm × 5 cm = £1.31, 10 cm × 10 cm = £2.48, 15 cm × 15 cm = £4.17, 15 cm × 20 cm = £5.70, 20 cm × 20 cm = £6.80, *with adhesive border*, 8 cm × 8 cm = £1.37, 10 cm × 10 cm = £2.10, 12.5 cm × 12.5 cm = £2.60, 17.5 cm × 17.5 cm = £5.20, 21 cm × 21 cm = £7.61, 25 cm × 30 cm = £9.85, 19.8 cm × 14 cm (heel) = £5.32, 20 cm × 16.9 cm (sacral) = £4.77

UrgoClean® (Urgo)

Pad, hydrocolloid fibres coated with soft-adherent lipo-colloidal wound contact layer, 6 cm × 6 cm = £0.94, 10 cm × 10 cm = £2.09, 15 cm × 20 cm = £3.93

Rope, non-woven rope containing hydrocolloid fibres, 2.5 cm × 40 cm = £2.35, 5 cm × 40 cm = £3.11

Versiva® **XC** (ConvaTec)

Hydrocolloid gelling foam dressing, without adhesive border, 7.5 cm × 7.5 cm = £1.39, 11 cm × 11 cm = £2.31, 15 cm × 15 cm = £4.26, 20 cm × 20 cm = £6.37; *with adhesive border*, 10 cm × 10 cm = £2.36, 14 cm × 14 cm = £3.19, 19 cm × 19 cm = £5.09, 22 cm × 22 cm = £5.65, 18.5 cm × 20.5 cm (heel) = £5.65, 21 cm × 25 cm (sacral) = £6.06

◢Polyurethane matrix dressing

Cutinova® **Hydro** (S&N Hlth.)

Polyurethane matrix with absorbent particles and waterproof polyurethane film, 5 cm × 6 cm = £1.19, 10 cm × 10 cm = £2.40, 15 cm × 20 cm = £5.07

A5.2.5   Foam dressings

Dressings containing hydrophilic polyurethane foam (adhesive or non-adhesive), with or without plastic film-backing, are suitable for all types of exuding wounds, but not for dry wounds; some foam dressings have a moisture-sensitive film backing with variable permeability dependant on the level of exudate

Foam dressings vary in their ability to absorb exudate; some are suitable only for lightly to moderately exuding wounds, others have greater fluid-handing capacity and are suitable for heavily exuding wounds. Saturated foam dressings can cause maceration of healthy skin if left in contact with the wound.

Foam dressings can be used in combination with other primary wound contact dressings. If used under compression bandaging or compression garments, the fluid-handling capacity of the foam dressing may be reduced. Foam dressings can also be used to provide a protective cushion for fragile skin. A foam dressing containing ibuprofen is available and may be useful for treating painful exuding wounds.

◢For lightly exuding wounds

Polyurethane Foam Film Dressing with Adhesive Border

PolyMem®, 5 cm × 5 cm = 50p (Aspen Medical)
Tielle® Lite, 11 cm × 11 cm = £2.28; 7 cm × 9 cm = £1.21; 8 cm × 15 cm = £2.81; 8 cm × 20 cm = £2.97 (Systagenix)

◢For lightly to moderately exuding wounds

Polyurethane Foam Dressing, BP 1993

Lyofoam®, 7.5 cm × 7.5 cm = £1.05, 10 cm × 10 cm = £1.20, 10 cm × 17.5 cm = £1.94, 15 cm × 20 cm = £2.61 (Mölnlycke)

Polyurethane Foam Film Dressing with Adhesive Border

Tielle®, 11 cm × 11 cm = £2.38; 15 cm × 15 cm = £3.89, 18 cm × 18 cm = £4.95, 7 cm × 9 cm = £1.28, 15 cm × 20 cm = £4.87, 18 cm × 18 cm (sacral) = £3.60 (Systagenix)

Polyurethane Foam Film Dressing without Adhesive Border

ActivHeal FlexiPore®, self-adhesive, 6 cm × 7 cm = 94p; 10 cm × 10 cm = £1.74, 15 cm × 20 cm = £3.70; 20 cm × 20 cm = £5.06; 10 cm × 30 cm = £3.63 (MedLogic)

Advazorb® Lite, 7.5 cm × 7.5 cm = £0.70, 10 cm × 10 cm = £0.97, 10 cm × 20 cm = £3.02, 12.5 cm × 12.5 cm = £1.43, 15 cm × 15 cm = £1.89, 20 cm × 20 cm = £3.38 (Advancis)

Allevyn® Lite, 5 cm × 5 cm = £1.06; 10 cm × 10 cm = £1.93; 10 cm × 20 cm = £3.31; 15 cm × 20 cm = £4.13 (S&N Hlth.)

Allevyn® Thin, self-adhesive, 5 cm × 6 cm = £1.00, 10 cm × 10 cm = £2.03, 15 cm × 15 cm = £3.35, 15 cm × 20 cm = £4.06 (S&N Hlth)

Kerraheel®, non-adhesive, 12 cm × 20 cm (heel) = £4.40 (Crawford)

PolyMem®, 7 cm × 7 cm (tube) = £1.70, 9 cm × 9 cm (tube) = £2.15, size 1 (finger/toe) = £2.50, size 2 (finger/toe) = £2.50, size 3 (finger/toe) = £2.50 (Aspen Medical)

Transorbent®, self-adhesive, 5 cm × 7 cm = £1.01; 10 cm × 10 cm = £1.90; 15 cm × 15 cm = £3.50; 20 cm × 20 cm = £5.59 (B. Braun)

UrgoCell® TLC, soft-adherent, 6 cm × 6 cm = £1.74, 10 cm × 10 cm = £2.53, 15 cm × 20 cm = £5.47, 12 cm × 19 cm (heel) = £4.52 (Urgo)

◀ For moderately to heavily exuding wounds

Polyurethane Foam Dressing

Cutimed® Cavity, 5 cm × 6 cm = £1.76, 10 cm × 10 cm = £2.92, 15 cm × 2 cm = £1.63, 15 cm × 15 cm = £4.39 (BSN Medical)

Kendall®, 5 cm × 5 cm = £0.71, 7.5 cm × 7.5 cm = £1.21, 10 cm × 10 cm = £1.06, 12.5 cm × 12.5 cm = £1.80, 15 cm × 15 cm = £2.60, 20 cm × 20 cm = £3.01, 10 cm × 20 cm = £2.05, 8.5 cm × 7.5 cm (fenestrated) = £0.91 (Covidien)

Polyurethane Foam Film Dressing with Adhesive Border

ActivHeal® Foam Adhesive, 7.5 cm × 7.5 cm = £1.18, 10 cm × 10 cm = £1.60, 12.5 cm × 12.5 cm = £1.68, 15 cm × 15 cm = £2.15, 20 cm × 20 cm = £4.42 (MedLogic)

Allevyn® Adhesive, 7.5 cm × 7.5 cm = £1.43, 10 cm × 10 cm = £2.10, 12.5 cm × 12.5 cm = £2.57, 17.5 cm × 17.5 cm = £5.07, 12.5 cm × 22.5 cm = £4.00, 22.5 cm × 22.5 cm = £7.38; (sacral) 17 cm × 17 cm = £3.80, 22 cm × 22 cm = £5.47 (S&N Hlth.)

Allevyn® Plus Adhesive, 12.5 cm × 12.5 cm = £3.16; 17.5 cm × 17.5 cm = £6.10; 12.5 cm × 22.5 cm = £5.60; (sacral) 17 cm × 17 cm = £4.61, 22 cm × 22 cm = £6.67 (S&N Hlth)

Biatain® Adhesive, 10 cm × 10 cm = £1.65 12.5 cm × 12.5 cm = £2.41, 18 cm × 18 cm = £4.86, 18 cm × 28 cm = £7.20, 23 cm × 23 cm (sacral) = £4.16, 19 cm × 20 cm (heel) = £4.85; 17 cm diameter (contour) = £4.67 (Coloplast)

Biatain® Silicone, 7.5 cm × 7.5 cm = £1.41, 10 cm × 10 cm = £2.27, 12.5 cm × 12.5 cm = £2.90, 15 cm × 15 cm = £3.98, 17.5 cm × 17.5 cm = £5.49 (Coloplast)

Kendall® Island, 10 cm × 10 cm = £1.51, 15 cm × 15 cm = £2.84, 20 cm × 20 cm = £5.36 (Coviden)

PermaFoam®, 16.5 cm × 18 cm (concave) = £ 3.82; 18 cm × 18 cm (sacral) = £3.14; 22 cm × 22 cm (sacral) = £3.61; *PermaFoam Comfort*® 8 cm × 8 cm = £1.06, 10 cm × 20 cm = £3.18, 11 cm × 11 cm = £2.02, 15 cm × 15 cm = £3.29, 20 cm × 20 cm = £4.78 (Hartmann)

PolyMem®, 5 cm × 7.6 cm = £1.12, 8.8 cm × 12.7 cm = £1.99, 10 cm × 13 cm = £2.11, 15 cm × 15 cm = £2.84, 16.5 cm × 20.9 cm = £6.54, 18.4 cm × 20 cm (sacral) = £4.39 (Aspen Medical)

Tegaderm® Foam Adhesive, 6.9 cm x 7.6 cm = £1.42, 10 cm × 11 cm = £2.33, 14.3 cm × 14.3 cm = £3.44, 14.3 cm × 15.6 cm = £4.12, 19 cm × 22.5 cm = £6.76, 6.9 cm x 6.9 cm (soft cloth border) = £1.66, 13.9 cm × 13.9 cm (heel) = £4.14 (3M)

Tielle® Plus, 11 cm × 11 cm = £2.63; 15 cm × 15 cm = £4.30; 15 cm × 20 cm = £5.39; 15 cm × 15 cm (sacrum) = £3.13; 20 cm × 26.5 cm (heel) = £4.45 (Systagenix)

Trufoam®, 11 cm × 11 cm = £2.18, 15 cm × 15 cm = £3.64, 7 cm × 9 cm = £1.14, 15 cm × 20 cm = £4.57 (Aspen Medical)

Polyurethane Foam Film Dressing without Adhesive Border

ActivHeal® Foam Non-Adhesive, 5 cm × 5 cm = £0.75, 10 cm × 10 cm = £1.13, 10 cm × 17.8 cm = £2.34, 10 cm × 20 cm =£2.34, 20 cm × 20 cm = £3.92, 18 cm × 12 cm (heel) = £3.48 (MedLogic)

Advazorb®, 5 cm × 5 cm = £0.65, 7.5 cm × 7.5 cm = £0.78, 10 cm × 10 cm = £1.08, 10 cm × 20 cm = £3.35, 12.5 cm × 12.5 cm = £1.59, 15 cm × 15 cm = £2.10, 20 cm × 20 cm = £3.75, 17 cm × 21 cm (heel) =£4.75 (Advancis)

Allevyn® Cavity, circular, 5 cm diameter = £3.97, 10 cm diameter = £9.46; tubular, 9 cm × 2.5 cm = £3.85, 12 cm × 4 cm = £6.78 (S&N Hlth.)

Allevyn® Compression, 5 cm × 6 cm = £1.18; 10 cm × 10 cm = £2.43; 15 cm × 15 cm = £4.12, 15 cm × 20 cm = £4.62 (S&N Hlth.)

Allevyn® Non-Adhesive, 5 cm × 5 cm = £1.21, 10 cm × 10 cm = £2.40, 10 cm × 20 cm = £3.86, 20 cm × 20 cm = £6.44, 10.5 cm × 13.5 cm (heel) = £4.81 (S&N Hlth.)

Allevyn® Plus Cavity, 5 cm × 6 cm = £1.78, 10 cm × 10 cm = £2.97, 15 cm × 20 cm = £5.95 (S&N Hlth.)

Askina® Foam, 10 cm × 10 cm = £2.10, 10 cm × 20 cm = £3.31, 20 cm × 20 cm = £5.53, 12 cm × 20 cm (heel) = £4.48; cavity dressing, 2.4 cm × 40 cm = £2.34 (B. Braun)

Biatain® -Ibu Non-Adhesive, impregnated with ibuprofen 0.5 mg/cm², 5 cm x 7 cm = £1.62, 10 cm x 12 cm = £3.12, 10 cm x 22.5 cm = £4.91, 15 cm x 15 cm = £4.91, 20 cm x 20 cm = £8.34 (Coloplast)
Note for cautions and contra-indications of ibuprofen see BNF section 10.1.1

Biatain® -Ibu Soft-Hold, impregnated with ibuprofen 0.5 mg/cm², 10 cm x 12 cm = £3.12, 10 cm x 22.5 cm = £4.91, 15 cm x 15 cm = £4.91 (Coloplast)
Note for cautions and contra-indications of ibuprofen see BNF section 10.1.1

Biatain® Non-Adhesive, 10 cm × 10 cm = £2.24, 10 cm × 20 cm = £3.70, 15 cm × 15 cm = £4.13, 20 cm × 20 cm = £6.13; 5 cm × 7 cm = £1.23; *Biatain® Soft-Hold*, 10 cm × 10 cm = £2.44, 15 cm × 15 cm = £4.05, 5 cm × 7 cm = £1.22, 10 cm × 20 cm = £3.70 (Coloplast)

Kendall® Plus, 5 cm × 5 cm = 80p, 7.5 cm × 7.5 cm = £1.39, 10 cm × 10 cm = £1.44, 15 cm × 15 cm = £3.32, 20 cm × 20 cm = £3.96, 10 cm × 20 cm = £2.64, 8.5 cm × 7.5 cm (fenestrated) = £1.22 (Covidien)

Kerraboot®, (clear or white), foot-shaped, extra small = £14.54, small = £14.83, large = £14.83, extra large = £14.54 (Crawford)

Lyofoam® Extra, 10 cm × 10 cm = £2.08, 17.5 cm × 10 cm = £3.52, 20 cm × 15 cm = £4.56 (Mölnlycke)

Lyofoam® Max, 7.5 cm × 8.5 cm = £1.05, 10 cm × 10 cm = £1.10, 10 cm × 20 cm = £1.94, 15 cm x 15 cm = £2.07, 15 cm × 20 cm = £2.61, 20 cm × 20 cm = £3.84 (Mölnlycke)

PermaFoam®, 10 cm × 10 cm = £2.02, 10 cm × 20 cm = £3.45, 15 cm × 15 cm = £3.82, 20 cm × 20 cm = £5.84; 6 cm diameter = £1.04, 8 cm × 8 cm (fenestrated) = £1.19; cavity dressing, 10 cm × 10 cm = £1.91 (Hartmann)

PolyMem®, 8 cm × 8 cm = £1.54, 10 cm × 10 cm = £2.39, 13 cm × 13 cm = £3.99, 17 cm × 19 cm = £5.90, 10 cm × 61 cm = £12.70, 20 cm × 60 cm = £30.55; *PolyMem®WIC* 8 cm × 8 cm (cavity) = £3.58; *PolyMem®Max* 11 cm × 11 cm = £2.88, 20 cm × 20 cm = £11.55 (Aspen Medical)

Tegaderm® Foam, 8.8 cm × 8.8 cm (fenestrated) = £2.17, 10 cm × 10 cm = £2.13, 10 cm × 20 cm = £3.61, 20 cm × 20 cm = £5.76, 10 cm × 60 cm = £12.19 (3M)

Tielle® Plus Borderless, 11 cm × 11 cm = £3.04; 15 cm × 20 cm = £5.51 (Systagenix)

Tielle® Xtra, 11 cm × 11 cm = £2.24; 15 cm × 15 cm = £3.37, 15 cm × 20 cm = £5.51 (Systagenix)

Trufoam® NA, 5 cm × 5 cm = £1.09, 10 cm × 10 cm = £2.07, 15 cm × 15 cm = £3.81 (Aspen Medical)

Cavi-Care® (S&N Hlth.)

Soft, conforming cavity wound dressing prepared by mixing thoroughly for 15 seconds immediately before use and allowing to expand its volume within the cavity. 20 g = £18.62

A5.2.6 Alginate dressings

Non-woven or fibrous, non-occlusive, alginate dressings, made from calcium alginate, or calcium sodium alginate, derived from brown seaweed, form a soft gel in contact with wound exudate.

Alginate dressings are highly absorbent and suitable for use on exuding wounds, and for the promotion of autolytic debridement of debris in very moist wounds. Alginate dressings also act as a haemostatic, but caution is needed because blood clots can cause the dressing to adhere to the wound surface. Alginate dressings should not be used if bleeding is heavy and extreme caution is needed if used for tumours with friable tissue.

Alginate sheets are suitable for use as a wound contact dressing for moderately to heavily exuding wounds and can be layered into deep wounds; alginate rope can be used in sinus and cavity wounds to improve absorption of exudate and prevent maceration. If the dressing does not have an adhesive border or integral adhesive plastic film backing, a secondary dressing will be required.

ActivHeal® (MedLogic)

Activheal® Alginate, calcium sodium alginate dressing, 5 cm × 5 cm = 58p, 10 cm × 10 cm = £1.13, 10 cm × 20 cm = £2.78; cavity dressing, 2 cm × 30 cm = £2.09

ActivHeal Aquafiber®, non-woven, calcium sodium alginate dressing, 5 cm × 5 cm = 74p, 10 cm × 10 cm = £1.77, 15 cm × 15 cm = £3.34; cavity dressing, 2 cm × 42 cm = £1.78

Algisite® M (S&N Hlth.)

Calcium alginate fibre, non-woven dressing, 5 cm × 5 cm = 87p, 10 cm × 10 cm = £1.80, 15 cm × 20 cm = £4.84; cavity dressing, 2 cm × 30 cm = £3.27

Algosteril® (S&N Hlth.)

Calcium alginate dressing. 5 cm × 5 cm = 87p, 10 cm × 10 cm = £1.98, 10 cm × 20 cm = £3.34; cavity dressing, 2 g, 30 cm = £3.57

Kaltostat® (ConvaTec)

Calcium alginate fibre, non-woven, 5 cm × 5 cm, = 90p, 7.5 cm × 12 cm = £1.96, 10 cm × 20 cm = £3.84, 15 cm × 25 cm = £6.61; cavity dressing, 2 g = £3.60

Kendall® (Covidien)

Calcium alginate dressing, 5 cm × 5 cm = 70p, 10 cm × 10 cm = £1.49, 10 cm × 14 cm = £2.41, 10 cm × 20 cm = £2.93, 15 cm × 25 cm = £5.15, 30 cm × 61 cm = £27.03; cavity dressing, 30 cm = £2.84, 61 cm = £4.98, 91 cm = £5.36

Kendall® Plus, calcium alginate dressing, 10 cm × 10 cm = £2.04

Kendall® Zn, calcium alginate and zinc dressing, 5 cm × 5 cm = 80p, 10 cm × 10 cm = £1.68, 10 cm × 20 cm = £3.30

Melgisorb® (Mölnlycke)

Calcium sodium alginate fibre, highly absorbent, gelling dressing, non-woven, 5 cm × 5 cm = 86p, 10 cm × 10 cm = £1.79, 10 cm × 20 cm = £3.36; cavity dressing, 32 cm × 2.2 cm, (2 g) = £3.39

SeaSorb® Soft (Coloplast)

Alginate and carboxymethylcellulose dressing, highly absorbent, gelling dressing, 5 cm × 5 cm = 91p, 10 cm × 10 cm = £2.18, 15 cm × 15 cm = £4.13; gelling filler, 44 cm = £2.57

Sorbalgon® (Hartmann)

Calcium alginate dressing, 5 cm × 5 cm = 77p, 10 cm × 10 cm = £1.62; *Sorbalgon® T*, cavity dressing, 2 g, 30 cm = £3.30

Sorbsan® (Aspen Medical)

Sorbsan® Flat, calcium alginate fibre, highly absorbent, flat non-woven pads, 5 cm × 5 cm = 80p, 10 cm × 10 cm = £1.68, 10 cm × 20 cm = £3.15

Sorbsan® Plus, alginate dressing bonded to a secondary absorbent viscose pad, 7.5 cm × 10 cm = £1.70, 10 cm × 15 cm = £3.01, 10 cm × 20 cm = £3.84, 15 cm × 20 cm = £5.33

Sorbsan® Ribbon, 40 cm (with probe) = £2.04

Sorbsan® Surgical Packing, 30 cm (2 g, with probe) = £3.47

Suprasorb® A (Activa)
Calcium alginate dressing, 5 cm × 5 cm = 59p, 10 cm × 10 cm = £1.16; cavity dressing, 30 cm (2 g) = £2.15

Tegaderm® Alginate (3M)
Calcium alginate dressing, 5 cm × 5 cm = 78p, 10 cm × 10 cm = £1.64; cavity dressing, 2 cm × 30.4 cm = £2.74

Urgosorb® (Urgo)
Alginate and carboxymethylcellulose dressing without adhesive border, 5 cm × 5 cm = 83p, 10 cm × 10 cm = £1.99, 10 cm × 20 cm = £3.64; cavity dressing, 30 cm = £2.65

A5.2.7 Capillary-action dressings

Capillary-action dressings consist of an absorbent core of hydrophilic fibres sandwiched between two low-adherent wound-contact layers to ensure no fibres are shed on to the wound surface. Wound exudate is taken up by the dressing and retained within the highly absorbent central layer.

The dressing may be applied intact to relatively superficial areas, but for deeper wounds or cavities it may be cut to shape to ensure good contact with the wound base. Multiple layers may be applied to heavily exuding wounds to further increase the fluid-absorbing capacity of the dressing. A secondary adhesive dressing is necessary.

Capillary-action dressings are suitable for use on all types of exuding wounds, but particularly on sloughy wounds where removal of fluid from the wound aids debridement; capillary-action dressings are contra-indicated for heavily bleeding wounds or arterial bleeding.

Advadraw® (Advancis)
Non-adherent dressing consisting of a soft viscose and polyester absorbent pad with central wicking layer between two perforated permeable wound contact layers. 5 cm × 7.5 cm = 57p, 10 cm × 10 cm = 88p, 10 cm × 15 cm = £1.19, 15 cm × 20 cm = £1.57
Advadraw Spiral®, 0.5 cm × 40 cm = 82p

Cerdak® Basic (CliniMed)
Non-adhesive wound contact sachet containing ceramic spheres, 5 cm × 5 cm = 70p, 10 cm × 10 cm = £1.56, 10 cm × 15 cm = £2.08; cavity dressing, 10 cm × 10 cm = £2.10, 10 cm × 15 cm = £2.63
Cerdak® Aerocloth, non-adhesive wound contact sachet containing ceramic spheres, with non-woven fabric adhesive backing, 5 cm × 5 cm = £1.37, 5 cm × 10 cm = £1.94
Cerdak® Aerofilm, non-adhesive wound contact sachet containing ceramic spheres, with waterproof transparent adhesive film backing, 5 cm × 5 cm = £1.51, 5 cm × 10 cm = £2.07

Sumar® (Lantor)
Sumar® Lite, for light to moderately exuding wounds and cavities, 5 cm × 5 cm = 93p, 10 cm × 10 cm = £1.59, 10 cm × 15 cm = £2.12
Sumar® Max, for heavily exuding wounds, 5 cm × 5 cm = 95p, 10 cm × 10 cm = £1.61, 10 cm × 15 cm = £2.15
Sumar®Spiral, 0.5 cm × 40 cm = £1.57

Vacutex® (Protex)
Low-adherent dressing consisting of two external polyester wound contact layers with central wicking polyester/cotton mix absorbent layer. 5 cm × 5 cm = 94p, 10 cm × 10 cm = £1.66, 10 cm × 15 cm = £2.23, 10 cm × 20 cm = £2.68, 15 cm × 20 cm = £3.14, 20 cm × 20 cm = £4.28

A5.2.8 Odour absorbent dressings

Dressings containing activated charcoal are used to absorb odour from wounds. The underlying cause of wound odour should be identified. Wound odour is most effectively reduced by debridement of slough, reduction in bacterial levels, and frequent dressing changes.

Fungating wounds and chronic infected wounds produce high volumes of exudate which can reduce the effectiveness of odour absorbent dressings. Many odour absorbent dressings are intended for use in combination with other dressings; odour absorbent dressings with a suitable wound contact layer can be used as a primary dressing.

Askina® Carbosorb (B. Braun)
Activated charcoal and non-woven viscose rayon dressing, 10 cm × 10 cm = £2.77, 10 cm × 20 cm = £5.34

CarboFLEX® (ConvaTec)
Dressing in 5 layers: wound-facing absorbent layer containing alginate and hydrocolloid; water-resistant second layer; third layer containing activated charcoal; non-woven absorbent fourth layer; water-resistant backing layer. 10 cm × 10 cm = £3.01, 8 cm × 15 cm = £3.61, 15 cm × 20 cm = £6.85

Carbopad® VC (Synergy Healthcare)
Activated charcoal non-absorbent dressing, 10 cm × 10 cm = £1.59, 10 cm × 20 cm = £2.15

CliniSorb® Odour Control Dressings (CliniMed)
Activated charcoal cloth enclosed in viscose rayon with outer polyamide coating. 10 cm × 10 cm = £1.78, 10 cm × 20 cm = £2.37, 15 cm × 25 cm = £3.81

Lyofoam® C (Medlock)
Lyofoam sheet with layer of activated charcoal cloth and additional outer envelope of polyurethane foam. 10 cm × 10 cm = £2.93, 15 cm × 20 cm = £6.65

Sorbsan® Plus Carbon (Aspen Medical)
Alginate dressing with activated carbon, 7.5 cm × 10 cm = £2.48, 10 cm × 15 cm = £4.81, 10 cm × 20 cm = £5.76, 15 cm × 20 cm = £6.63

A5.3 Antimicrobial dressings

Spreading infection at the wound site requires treatment with systemic antibacterials.

For local wound infection, a topical antimicrobial dressing can be used to reduce the level of bacteria at the wound surface but will not eliminate a spreading infection. Some dressings are designed to release the antimicrobial into the wound, others act upon the bacteria after absorption from the wound. The amount of exudate present and the level of infection should be taken into account when selecting an antimicrobial dressing.

Medical grade honey (section A5.3.1), has anti-microbial and anti-inflammatory properties. Dressings impregnated with iodine (section A5.3.2), can be used to treat clinically infected wounds. Dressings containing silver (section A5.3.3), should be used only when clinical signs or symptoms of infection are present.

Dressings containing other antimicrobials (section A5.3.4) such as polihexanide (polyhexamethylene biguanide) or dialkylcarbamoyl chloride are available for use on infected wounds. Although hypersensitivity is unlikely with chlorhexidine impregnated tulle dressing, the antibacterial efficacy of these dressings has not been established.

A5.3.1 Honey

Medical grade honey has antimicrobial and anti-inflammatory properties and can be used for acute or chronic wounds. Medical grade honey has osmotic properties, producing an environment that promotes autolytic debridement; it can help control wound malodour. Honey dressings should not be used on patients with extreme sensitivity to honey, bee stings or bee products. Patients with diabetes should be monitored for changes in blood-glucose concentrations during treatment with topical honey or honey-impregnated dressings.

◢ Sheet dressing

Actilite® (Advancis)
Knitted viscose impregnated with medical grade manuka honey and manuka oil, 10 cm × 10 cm = 97p, 10 cm × 20 cm = £1.88

Activon Tulle® (Advancis)
Knitted viscose impregnated with medical grade manuka honey, 5 cm × 5 cm = £1.82, 10 cm × 10 cm = £3.06
Where no size stated by the prescriber the 5 cm size to be supplied

Algivon® (Advancis)
Absorbent, non-adherent calcium alginate dressing impregnated with medical grade manuka honey, 5 cm × 5 cm = £2.13, 10 cm × 10 cm = £3.59
Algivon® Plus, reinforced calcium alginate dressing impregnated with medical grade manuka honey, 5 cm × 5 cm = £1.96, 10 cm × 10 cm = £3.36, 2.5 cm × 20 cm (ribbon with with probe) = £3.36

Medihoney® (Medihoney)
Antibacterial Honey Tulle, woven fabric impregnated with medical grade manuka honey, 10 cm × 10 cm = £2.98
Gel sheet, sodium alginate dressing impregnated with medical grade honey, 5 cm × 5 cm = £1.75, 10 cm × 10 cm = £4.20
Antibacterial Honey Apinate®, non-adherent calcium alginate dressing, impregnated with medical grade honey, 10 cm × 10 cm = £5.09

Melladerm® Plus Tulle (Danetre)
Knitted viscose impregnated with medical grade honey (Bulgarian, mountain flower) 45% in a basis containing polyethylene glycol, 10 cm × 10 cm = £2.10

MelMax® (CliniMed)
Acetate wound contact layer impregnated with buckwheat honey 75% in ointment basis, 5 cm × 6 cm = £4.82, 8 cm × 10 cm = £9.90, 8 cm × 20 cm = £19.79

Mesitran® (Aspen Medical)
Hydrogel, semi-permeable dressing impregnated with medical grade honey, 10 cm × 10 cm = £2.55, 15 cm × 20 cm = £5.31; with adhesive border, 10 cm × 10 cm = £2.66, 15 cm × 13 cm (sacral) = £4.50, 15 cm × 15 cm = £4.70
Mesitran® Mesh, hydrogel, non-adherent wound contact layer, without adhesive border, 10 cm × 10 cm = £2.45

◢ Honey-based topical application
Medical grade honey is applied directly to the wound and covered with a primary low adherence wound dressing; an additional secondary dressing may be required for exuding wounds.

Activon® (Advancis)
Honey, (medical grade, manuka), 25-g tube = £2.02

MANUKApli® (Manuka Medical)
Honey, (medical grade, manuka), 15-g tube = £2.95

Medihoney® (Medihoney)
Antibacterial Medical Honey, honey (medical grade, Leptospermum sp.), 20-g tube = £3.96, 50-g tube = £9.90
Antibacterial Wound Gel, honey (medical grade, Leptospermum sp.), 80% in natural waxes and oils, 10-g tube = £2.69, 20-g tube = £4.02
Note Antibacterial Wound Gel is not recommended for use in deep wounds or body cavities where removal of waxes may be difficult

Melladerm® Plus (Danetre)
Honey, (medical grade; Bulgarian, mountain flower) 45% in basis containing polyethylene glycol, 20-g tube = £4.49, 50-g tube = £8.50

Mesitran® (Aspen Medical)
Ointment, honey (medical grade) 47%, 15-g tube = £3.47, 50-g tube = £9.55
Excipients include lanolinOintment S, honey (medical grade) 40%, 15-g tube = £3.46
Excipients include lanolin

A5.3.2 Iodine

Cadexomer–iodine, like povidone–iodine, releases free iodine when exposed to wound exudate. The free iodine acts as an antiseptic on the wound surface, the cadexomer absorbs wound exudate and encourages de-sloughing.

Two-component hydrogel dressings containing glucose oxidase and iodide ions generate a low level of free iodine in the presence of moisture and oxygen.

Povidone–iodine fabric dressing is a knitted viscose dressing with povidone–iodine incorporated in a hydrophilic polyethylene glycol basis; this facilitates diffusion of the iodine into the wound and permits removal of the dressing by irrigation. The iodine has a wide spectrum of antimicrobial activity but it is rapidly deactivated by wound exudate.

Systemic absorption of iodine may occur, particularly from large wounds or with prolonged use.

Iodoflex® (S&N Hlth.)

Paste, iodine 0.9% as cadexomer–iodine in a paste basis with gauze backing, 5-g unit = £3.88; 10 g = £7.76; 17 g = £12.29

Uses   for treatment of chronic exuding wounds; max. single application 50 g, max. weekly application 150 g; max. duration up to 3 months in any single course of treatment

Cautions   iodine may be absorbed, particularly from large wounds or during prolonged use; severe renal impairment; history of thyroid disorder

Contra-indications   children; patients receiving lithium; thyroid disorders; pregnancy and breast-feeding

Iodosorb® (S&N Hlth.)

Ointment, iodine 0.9% as cadexomer–iodine in an ointment basis, 10 g = £4.29; 20 g = £8.58

Powder, iodine 0.9% as cadexomer–iodine microbeads, 3-g sachet = £1.84

Uses   for treatment of chronic exuding wounds; max. single application 50 g, max. weekly application 150 g; max. duration up to 3 months in any single course of treatment

Cautions   iodine may be absorbed, particularly from large wounds or during prolonged use; severe renal impairment; history of thyroid disorder

Contra-indications   children; patients receiving lithium; thyroid disorders; pregnancy and breast-feeding

Iodozyme® (Archimed)

Hydrogel (two-component dressing containing glucose oxidase and iodide ions), 6.5 cm × 5 cm = £7.50, 10 cm × 10 cm = £12.50

Uses   antimicrobial dressing for lightly to moderately exuding wounds

Cautions   children; pregnancy and breast-feeding

Contra-indications   thyroid disorders; patients receiving lithium

Oxyzyme® (Archimed)

Hydrogel (two-component dressing containing glucose oxidase and iodide ions), 6.5 cm × 5 cm = £6.00, 10 cm × 10 cm = £10.00

Uses   non-infected, dry to moderately exuding wounds

Cautions   children; pregnancy and breast-feeding

Contra-indications   thyroid disorders; patients receiving lithium

Povidone–iodine Fabric Dressing

(Drug Tariff specification 43). Knitted viscose primary dressing impregnated with povidone–iodine ointment 10%, 5 cm × 5 cm = 32p; 9.5 cm × 9.5 cm = 48p (Systagenix—*Inadine®*)

Uses   wound contact layer for abrasions and superficial burns

Cautions   iodine may be absorbed particularly if large wounds treated; children under 6 months; thyroid disease

Contra-indications   severe renal impairment; pregnancy; breast-feeding

A5.3.3 Silver

Antimicrobial dressings containing **silver** should be used only when infection is suspected as a result of clinical signs or symptoms (see also p. 46). Silver ions exert an antimicrobial effect in the presence of wound exudate; the volume of wound exudate as well as the presence of infection should be considered when selecting a silver-containing dressing. Silver-impregnated dressings should not be used routinely for the management of uncomplicated ulcers. It is recommended that

these dressings should not be used on acute wounds as there is some evidence to suggest they delay wound healing.

Dressings impregnated with silver sulfadiazine have broad antimicrobial activity; if silver sulfadiazine is applied to large areas, or used for prolonged periods, there is a risk of blood disorders and skin discoloration (see BNF section 13.10.1.1). The use of silver sulfadiazine-impregnated dressings is contra-indicated in neonates, in pregnancy, and in patients with significant renal or hepatic impairment, sensitivity to sulphonamides, or G6PD deficiency. Large amounts of silver sulfadiazine applied topically may interact with other drugs—see Appendix 1 (sulfonamides).

◢ **Low adherence dressings**

Acticoat® (S&N Hlth.)

Three-layer antimicrobial barrier dressing consisting of a polyester core between low adherent silver-coated high density polyethylene mesh (for 3-day wear), 5 cm × 5 cm = £3.30, 10 cm × 10 cm = £8.07, 10 cm × 20 cm = £12.62, 20 cm × 40 cm = £43.18

Acticoat® 7 five-layer antimicrobial barrier dressing consisting of a polyester core between low adherent silver-coated high density polyethylene mesh (for 7-day wear), 5 cm × 5 cm = £5.74, 10 cm × 12.5 cm = £17.11, 15 cm × 15 cm = £30.76

Acticoat® Flex 3, conformable antimicrobial barrier dressing consisting of a polyester core between low adherent silver-coated high density polyethylene mesh (for 3-day wear), 5 cm × 5 cm = £3.32, 10 cm × 10 cm = £8.10, 10 cm × 20 cm = £12.66, 20 cm × 40 cm = £43.34

Acticoat® Flex 7, conformable antimicrobial barrier dressing consisting of a polyester core between low adherent silver-coated high density polyethylene mesh (for 7-day wear), 5 cm × 5 cm = £5.77, 15 cm × 15 cm = £30.88, 10 cm × 12.5 cm = £17.18

Atrauman® Ag (Hartmann)

Non-adherent polyamide fabric impregnated with silver and neutral triglycerides, 5 cm × 5 cm = 49p, 10 cm × 10 cm = £1.19, 10 cm × 20 cm = £2.32

◢ **With charcoal**

Actisorb® Silver 220 (Systagenix)

Knitted fabric of activated charcoal, with one-way stretch, with silver residues, within spun-bonded nylon sleeve. 6.5 cm × 9.5 cm = £1.64, 10.5 cm × 10.5 cm = £2.58, 10.5 cm × 19 cm = £4.70

◢ **Soft polymer dressings**

Allevyn® Ag Gentle (S&N Hlth.)

Soft polymer wound contact dressing, with silver sulfadiazine impregnated polyurethane foam layer, *with adhesive border*, 7.5 cm × 7.5 cm = £3.99, 10 cm × 10 cm = £5.99, 12.5 cm × 12.5 cm = £7.71, 17.5 cm × 17.5 cm = £14.69; *without adhesive border*, 5 cm × 5 cm = £3.12, 10 cm × 10 cm = £5.82, 10 cm × 20 cm = £9.62, 15 cm × 15 cm = £10.83, 20 cm × 20 cm = £16.04

Contra-indications   see notes above

Mepilex® Ag (Mölnlycke)
Soft silicone wound contact dressing with polyurethane foam film backing, with silver, *with adhesive border*, 7 cm × 7.5 cm = £3.30, 10 cm × 12.5 cm = £5.97, 10 cm × 20 cm = £8.69, 10 cm × 25 cm = £10.88, 10 cm × 30 cm = £13.04, 15 cm × 17.5 cm = £10.96, 17 cm × 20 cm = £14.20, 18 cm × 18 cm (sacral) = £11.46, 20 cm × 20 cm (sacral) = £13.93, 23 cm × 23 cm = £18.30; *without adhesive border*, 10 cm × 10 cm = £5.91, 10 cm × 20 cm = £9.75, 15 cm × 15 cm = £10.98, 20 cm × 20 cm = £16.27, 20 cm × 50 cm = £61.22, 13 cm × 20 cm (heel) = £12.38, 15 cm × 22 cm = £13.87

Urgotul® Silver (Urgo)
Non-adherent soft polymer wound contact dressing, with silver, 10 cm × 12 cm = £3.34, 15 cm × 20 cm = £9.09

Urgotul® Duo Silver, non-adherent, soft polymer wound contact dressing, with silver, 5 cm × 7 cm = £1.95, 11 cm × 11 cm = £3.87, 15 cm × 20 cm = £9.35

Urgotul® SSD (Urgo)
Non-adherent, soft polymer wound contact dressing, with silver sulfadiazine, 11 cm × 11 cm = £2.99, 16 cm × 21 cm = £8.48
Contra-indications see notes above

◀ Hydrocolloid dressings

Aquacel® Ag (ConvaTec)
Soft non-woven pad containing hydrocolloid fibres, (silver impregnated), 4 cm × 10 cm = £2.70, 4 cm × 20 cm = £3.52, 4 cm × 30 cm = £5.27, 5 cm × 5 cm = £1.86, 10 cm × 10 cm = £4.44, 15 cm × 15 cm = £8.36, 20 cm × 30 cm = £20.73; 1 cm × 45 cm (ribbon) = £2.97, 2 cm × 45 cm (ribbon) = £4.46

Biatain® Ag Hydrocolloid (Coloplast)
Semi-permeable, antimicrobial barrier dressing with ionic silver (silver sodium thiosulphate), 10 cm × 10 cm = £6.72, 15 cm × 15 cm = £13.44

Physiotulle® Ag (Coloplast)
Non-adherent polyester fabric with hydrocolloid and silver sulfadiazine, 10 cm × 10 cm = £2.14
Contra-indications see notes above

◀ Foam dressings

Acticoat® Moisture Control (S&N Hlth.)
Three layer polyurethane dressing consisting of a silver coated layer, a foam layer, and a waterproof layer, 5 cm × 5 cm = £6.76, 10 cm × 10 cm = £15.82, 10 cm × 20 cm = £30.82

Allevyn® Ag (S&N Hlth.)
Silver sulfadiazine impregnated polyurethane foam film dressing *with adhesive border*, 7.5 cm × 7.5 cm = £3.27, 10 cm × 10 cm = £5.16, 12.5 cm × 12.5 cm = £6.78, 17.5 cm × 17.5 cm = £13.03, 17 cm × 17 cm (sacral) = £10.18, 22 cm × 22 cm (sacral) = £13.64; *without adhesive border*, 5 cm × 5 cm = £3.06, 10 cm × 10 cm = £5.76, 15 cm × 15 cm = £10.91, 20 cm × 20 cm = £15.99, 10.5 cm × 13.5 cm (heel) = £10.09
Contra-indications see notes above

Biatain® Ag (Coloplast)
Silver impregnated polyurethane foam film dressing *with adhesive border*, 12.5 cm × 12.5 cm = £8.71, 18 cm × 18 cm = £17.47, 19 cm × 20 cm (heel) = £17.23, 23 cm × 23 cm (sacral) = £18.31; *without adhesive border*, 10 cm × 10 cm = £7.61, 5 cm × 7 cm = £3.13, 10 cm × 20 cm = £13.99, 15 cm × 15 cm = £15.28, 20 cm × 20 cm = £21.55; 5 cm × 8 cm (cavity) = £3.79

PolyMem® Silver (Aspen Medical)
Silver impregnated polyurethane foam film dressing, *with adhesive border*, 5 cm × 7.6 cm (oval) = £2.20, 12.7 cm × 8.8 cm (oval) = £5.43; *without adhesive border*, 10.8 cm × 10.8 cm = £8.60, 17 cm × 19 cm = £17.22; 8 cm × 8 cm (cavity) = £6.84

UrgoCell® Silver (Urgo)
Non-adherent, polyurethane foam film dressing with silver in wound contact layer, 6 cm × 6 cm = £4.11, 10 cm × 10 cm = £5.65, 15 cm × 20 cm = £10.17

◀ Alginate dressings

Acticoat® Absorbent (S&N Hlth.)
Calcium alginate dressing with a silver coated antimicrobial barrier, 5 cm × 5 cm = £5.04, 10 cm × 12.5 cm = £12.11; 2 cm × 30 cm (cavity) = £12.18

Algisite® Ag (S&N Hlth.)
Calcium alginate dressing, with silver, 5 cm × 5 cm = £1.56, 10 cm × 10 cm = £3.90, 10 cm × 20 cm = £7.17; 2 g, 30 cm (cavity) = £5.38

Melgisorb® Ag (Mölnlycke)
Alginate and carboxymethylcellulose dressing, with ionic silver, 5 cm × 5 cm = £1.71, 10 cm × 10 cm = £3.43, 15 cm × 15 cm = £7.25; 3 cm × 44 cm (cavity) = £4.32

Seasorb® Ag (Coloplast)
Alginate and carboxymethylcellulose dressing, with ionic silver, 5 cm × 5 cm = £1.53, 10 cm × 10 cm = £3.74, 15 cm × 15 cm = £6.12; 3 cm × 44 cm (cavity) = £4.05

Silvercel® (Systagenix)
Alginate and carboxymethylcellulose dressing impregnated with silver, 2.5 cm × 30.5 cm = £4.45, 5 cm × 5 cm = £1.68, 10 cm × 20 cm = £7.68, 11 cm × 11 cm = £4.14

Silvercel® Non-adherent, alginate and carboxymethylcellulose dressing with film wound contact layer, impregnated with silver, 5 cm × 5 cm = £1.62, 11 cm × 11 cm = £3.89, 10 cm × 20 cm = £7.25; 2.5 cm × 30.5 cm (cavity) = £3.94

Sorbsan® Silver (Aspen Medical)
Sorbsan® Silver Flat, calcium alginate fibre, highly absorbent, flat non-woven pads, with silver, 5 cm × 5 cm = £1.57, 10 cm × 10 cm = £3.97, 10 cm × 20 cm = £7.26

Sorbsan® Silver Plus, calcium alginate dressing with absorbent backing, with silver, 7.5 cm × 10 cm = £3.31, 10 cm × 15 cm = £5.50, 10 cm × 20 cm = £6.69, 15 cm × 20 cm = £8.98

Sorbsan® Silver Plus SA, calcium alginate dressing with absorbent backing and adhesive border, with silver, 11.5 cm × 14 cm = £5.38, 14 cm × 19 cm = £7.73, 14 cm × 24 cm = £8.51, 19 cm × 24 cm = £9.49

Sorbsan® Silver Ribbon, with silver, 40 cm (with probe) = £4.15

Sorbsan® Silver Surgical Packing, with silver, 30 cm (2 g, with probe) = £5.76

Suprasorb® A + Ag (Activa)
Calcium alginate dressing, with silver, 5 cm × 5 cm = £1.54, 10 cm × 10 cm = £3.87, 10 cm × 20 cm = £7.14; cavity dressing, 30 cm (2 g) = £5.72

Tegaderm® Alginate Ag (3M)
Calcium alginate and carboxymethylcellulose dressing, with silver, 5 cm × 5 cm = £1.35, 10 cm × 10 cm = £3.15; cavity dressing 3 cm × 30 cm = £3.60

Urgosorb®Silver (Urgo)
Alginate and carboxymethylcellulose dressing, impregnated with silver, 5 cm × 5 cm = £1.44, 10 cm × 10 cm = £3.44, 10 cm × 20 cm = £6.48; cavity dressing, 2.5 cm × 30 cm = £3.46

A5.3.4 Other antimicrobials

Chlorhexidine Gauze Dressing, BP 1993 ◢
Fabric of leno weave, weft and warp threads of cotton and/or viscose yarn, impregnated with ointment containing chlorhexidine acetate, 5 cm × 5 cm = 28p; 10 cm × 10 cm = 58p (S&N Hlth.—*Bactigras®*)

Cutimed® Sorbact (BSN Medical)
Low adherence acetate tissue impregnated with dialkylcarbamoyl chloride, (dressing pad) 7 cm × 9 cm = £3.30, 10 cm × 10 cm = £5.16, 10 cm × 20 cm = £8.04; (swabs) 4 cm × 6 cm = £1.55, 7 cm × 9 cm = £2.58, (round swabs) 3 cm, 5 pad pack = £3.09; (ribbon gauze, cotton) 2 cm × 50 cm = £3.78, 5 cm × 2 m = £7.45

Gel, hydrogel dressing impregnated with dialkylcarbamoyl chloride, 7.5 cm × 7.5 cm = £2.49, 7.5 cm × 15 cm = £4.20

Cutimed® Sorbact Hydroactive, non-adhesive gel dressing with hydropolymer matrix and acetate fabric coated with dialkylcarbamoyl chloride, 7 cm × 8.5 cm = £3.57, 14 cm × 14 cm = £5.21, 14 cm × 24 cm = £8.35, 19 cm × 19 cm = £9.81, 24 cm × 24 cm = £14.87

Cutimed® Sorbact Hydroactive B, gel dressing with hydropolymer matrix and acetate fabric coated with dialkylcarbamoyl chloride, with adhesive border, 5 cm × 6.5 cm = £3.86, 10 cm × 10 cm =£6.88, 10 cm × 20 cm = £11.02, 15 cm × 15 cm = £12.95, 20 cm × 20 cm = £19.63

Flaminal® (Crawford)
Forte gel, alginate with glucose oxidase and lactoperoxidase, for moderately to heavily exuding wounds, 15 g = £7.26, 50 g = £24.04

Hydro gel, alginate with glucose oxidase and lactoperoxidase, for lightly to moderately exuding wounds, 15 g = £7.26, 50 g = £24.04

Kendall AMD® (Covidien)
Foam dressing with polihexanide, *without adhesive border*, 5 cm × 5 cm = £2.45, 10 cm × 10 cm = £4.62, 15 cm × 15 cm = £8.75, 20 cm × 20 cm = £12.82, 8.8 cm × 7.5 cm (fenestrated) = £4.15, 10 cm × 20 cm = £8.75

Kendall AMD® Plus 10 cm × 10 cm = £4.85, 8.8 cm × 7.5 cm (fenestrated) = £4.35

Octenilin® (Schülke)
Wound gel, hydroxyethylcellulose and propylene glycol, with octenidine hydrochloride, 20 mL = £4.78

Prontosan® Wound Gel (B. Braun)
Hydrogel containing betaine surfactant and polihexanide, 30 mL = £6.12

Suprasorb® X + PHMB (Activa)
Biosynthetic cellulose fibre dressing with polihexanide, 5 cm × 5 cm = £2.42, 9 cm × 9 cm = £4.81, 14 cm × 20 cm = £10.95; 2 cm × 21 cm (rope) = £6.82

Telfa® AMD (Covidien)
Low adherence absorbent perforated plastic film faced dressing with polihexanide, 7.5 cm × 10 cm = 17p, 7.5 cm × 20 cm = 28p

Telfa® AMD Island, low adherence dressing with adhesive border and absorbent pad, with polihexanide, 10 cm × 12.5 cm = 58p, 10 cm × 20 cm = 85p, 10 cm × 25.5 cm = 96p, 10 cm × 35 cm = £1.19

◢Irrigation fluids

Octenilin® (Schülke)
Wound irrigation solution, aqueous solution containing glycerol, ethylhexylglycerin and octenidine hydrochloride, 350 mL = £4.60

Prontosan® Wound Irrigation Solution (B.Braun)
Aqueous solution containing betaine surfactant and polihexanide, 40 mL = £0.58, 350 mL = £4.66

A5.4 Specialised dressings

A5.4.1 Protease-modulating matrix dressings

Protease-modulating matrix dressings alter the activity of *proteolytic enzymes* in chronic wounds; the clinical significance of this approach is yet to be demonstrated.

Cadesorb® (S&N Hlth.)
Ointment, starch-based, 10 g = £5.10, 20 g = £8.69

Catrix® (Cranage)
Powder, collagen matrix (cartilage, bovine), 1-g sachet = £3.80

Promogran® (Systagenix)
Collagen and oxidised regenerated cellulose matrix, applied directly to wound and covered with suitable dressing, 28 cm^2 (hexagonal) = £5.19, 123 cm^2 (hexagonal) = £15.62

Promogran® Prisma® Matrix, collagen, silver and oxidised regenerated cellulose matrix, applied directly to wound and covered with suitable dressing, 28 cm^2 (hexagonal) = £6.31, 123 cm^2 (hexagonal) = £17.98

Tegaderm® Matrix (3M)

Cellulose acetate matrix, impregnated with polyhydrated ionogens ointment in polyethylene glycol basis, 5 cm × 6 cm = £4.75, 8 cm × 10 cm = £9.75

UrgoStart® (Urgo)

Soft adherent polymer matrix containing nano-oligosaccharide factor (NOSF), with polyurethane foam film backing, 6 cm × 6 cm = £4.30, 10 cm × 10 cm = £5.95, 15 cm × 20 cm = £10.70, 12 cm × 19 cm (heel) = £8.20

UrgoStart® Contact (Urgo)

Non-adherent soft polymer wound contact dressing containing nano-oligosaccharide factor (NOSF), 5 cm × 7 cm = £2.80, 11 cm × 11 cm = £3.98, 16 cm × 21 cm = £9.50

Xelma® (Mölnlycke)

Gel, alginate and propylene glycol with extracellular matrix proteins (amelogenins), 0.5-mL syringe = £56.98, 1-mL syringe = £99.72

A5.4.2 Silicone keloid dressings

Silicone gel and gel sheets are used to reduce or prevent hypertrophic and keloid scarring. They should not be used on open wounds. Application times should be increased gradually. Silicone sheets can be washed and reused.

◀Silicone sheets

Advasil® Conform (Advancis)

Self-adhesive silicone gel sheet with polyurethane film backing, 10 cm × 10 cm = £5.20, 10 cm × 15 cm = £9.17

BAP Scar Care T® (BAP)

Self-adhesive silicone gel sheet, 5 cm × 7 cm = £3.15, 5 cm × 30 cm = £9.00, 10 cm × 15 cm = £9.00

Cica-Care® (S&N Hlth.)

Soft, self-adhesive, semi-occlusive silicone gel sheet with backing. 6 cm × 12 cm = £13.79; 15 cm × 12 cm = £26.89

Ciltech® (Su-Med)

Silicone gel sheet, 10 cm × 10 cm = £7.50, 15 cm × 15 cm = £14.00, 10 cm × 20 cm = £12.50

Dermatix® (Meda)

Self-adhesive silicone gel sheet (clear- or fabric-backed), 4 cm × 13 cm = £6.69, 13 cm × 13 cm = £15.34, 13 cm × 25 cm = £27.73, 20 cm × 30 cm = £50.49

Mepiform® (Mölnlycke)

Self-adhesive silicone gel sheet with polyurethane film backing, 5 cm × 7 cm = £3.26, 9 cm × 18 cm = £12.76, 4 cm × 31 cm = £10.31

Scar FX® (Jobskin)

Self-adhesive, transparent, silicone gel sheet, 10 cm × 20 cm = £16.00, 25.5 cm × 30.5 cm = £60.00, 3.75 cm × 22.5 cm = £12.00, 7.5 cm diameter = £8.50, 22.5 cm × 14.5 cm = £12.00

Silgel® (Nagor)

Silicone gel sheet, 10 cm × 10 cm = £13.50; 20 cm × 20 cm = £40.00; 40 cm × 40 cm = £144.00; 10 cm × 5 cm = £7.50; 15 cm x 10 cm = £19.50; 30 cm × 5 cm = £19.50; 10 cm × 30 cm = £31.50; 25 cm × 15 cm (submammary) = £21.12; 46 cm × 8.5 cm (abdominal) = £39.46; 5.5 cm diameter (circular) = £4.00

◀Silicone gel

BAP Scar Care® (BAP)

Silicone gel, 20 g = £17.00

Ciltech® (Su-Med)

Silicone gel, 15 g = £17.50, 60 g = £50.00

Dermatix® (Meda)

Silicone gel, 15 g = £16.18, 60 g = £58.81

Kelo-cote® (Sinclair IS)

Silicone gel, 15 g = £17.88, 60 g = £51.00

Silicone spray, 100 mL = £51.00

NewGel+®E (Advantech Surgical)

Silicone gel with vitamin E, 15 g = £17.70

ScarSil® (Jobskin)

Silicone gel, 30 g = £15.00

Silgel® STC-SE (Nagor)

Silicone gel, 20-mL tube = £19.00

A5.5 Adjunct dressings and appliances

A5.5.1 Surgical absorbents

Surgical absorbents applied directly to the wound have many disadvantages—dehydration of and adherence to the wound, shedding of fibres, and the leakage of exudate ('strike through') with an associated risk of infection. Gauze and cotton absorbent dressings can be used as secondary layers in the management of heavily exuding wounds (but see also Capillary-action dressings, section A5.2.7). Absorbent cotton gauze fabric can be used for swabbing and cleaning skin. Ribbon gauze can be used post-operatively to pack wound cavities, but adherence to the wound bed will cause bleeding and tissue damage on removal of the dressing—an advanced wound dressing (e.g. hydrocolloid-fibrous (section A5.2.4), foam (section A5.2.5), or alginate (section A5.2.6)) layered into the cavity is often more suitable.

◀Cotton

Absorbent Cotton, BP

Carded cotton fibres of not less than 10 mm average staple length, available in rolls and balls, 25 g = 72p; 100 g = £1.64; 500 g = £5.53 (most suppliers).

Drug Tariff specifies 25-g pack to be supplied when weight not stated

Absorbent Cotton, Hospital Quality

As for absorbent cotton but lower quality materials, shorter staple length etc. 100 g = £1.14; 500 g = £3.60 (most suppliers)

Drug Tariff specifies to be supplied only where specifically ordered

Note Not suitable for wound cleansing

◢Gauze and tissue

Absorbent Cotton Gauze, BP 1988
Cotton fabric of plain weave, in rolls and as swabs
(see below), usually Type 13 light, sterile, 90 cm (all)
× 1 m = £1.08; 3 m = £2.26; 5 m = £3.52; 10 m =
£6.73 (most suppliers). 1-m packet supplied when
no size stated
Note Drug Tariff also includes unsterilised absorbent cotton
gauze, 25 m roll = £15.42

**Absorbent Cotton and Viscose Ribbon Gauze, BP
1988**
Woven fabric in ribbon form with fast selvedge
edges, warp threads of cotton, weft threads of
viscose or combined cotton and viscose yarn,
sterile. 5 m (both) × 1.25 cm = 81p; 2.5 cm = 90p

Gauze and Cotton Tissue, BP 1988
Consists of absorbent cotton enclosed in absorbent
cotton gauze type 12 or absorbent cotton and
viscose gauze type 2. 500 g = £7.01 (most suppliers,
including Robinsons—*Gamgee Tissue*® (blue label))

Gauze and Cotton Tissue
(Drug Tariff specification 14). Similar to above.
500 g = £5.12 (most suppliers, including
Robinsons—*Gamgee Tissue*® (pink label))
Drug Tariff specifies to be supplied only where specifically
ordered

◢Lint

Absorbent Lint, BPC ◢
Cotton cloth of plain weave with nap raised on one
side from warp yarns. 25 g = 89p; 100 g = £2.74;
500 g = £11.52 (most suppliers).
Drug Tariff specifies 25-g pack supplied where no quantity
stated
Note Not recommended for wound management

◢Pads

Absorbent Dressing Pads, Sterile
Drisorb®, 10 cm × 20 cm = 17p (Synergy
Healthcare)
PremierPad®, 10 cm × 20 cm = 18p, 20 cm ×
20 cm = 25p (Shermond)
Xupad®, 10 cm × 20 cm = 17p, 20 cm × 20 cm =
28p, 20 cm × 40 cm = 40p (Richardson)

[1]Surgipad® (Systagenix) ⒿⒽⓈ
Absorbent pad of absorbent cotton and viscose in
sleeve of non-woven viscose fabric, pouch 12 cm ×
10 cm = 18p, 20 cm × 10 cm = 25p, 20 cm ×
20 cm = 30p, 40 cm × 20 cm = 41p; *non sterile* pack
12 cm × 10 cm = 5p, 20 cm × 10 cm = 10p, 20 cm
× 20 cm = 17p, 40 cm × 20 cm = 28p

A5.5.2 Wound drainage pouches

Wound drainage pouches can be used in the management of wounds and fistulas with significant levels of
exudate.

Biotrol® (B. Braun)
Draina S Fistula, wound drainage pouch, mini (cut
to 20 mm), 150-mL capacity = £2.44; medium (cut
to 50 mm), 350-mL capacity = £3.64; large (cut to
88 mm), 500-mL capacity = £4.48

Draina S Vision, wound drainage pouch, (cut to
50 mm), 150-mL capacity = £9.39; (cut to 88 mm),
250-mL capacity = £9.92; (cut to 100 mm), 300-mL
capacity = £11.51

Dermasure® (ADI Medical)
Pouch, small (wound size up to 9 cm × 16 cm) =
£15.60; medium (wound size up to 15 cm × 27 cm)
= £20.80

Eakin® (Eakin)
Wound pouch, *fold and tuck closure*, small (wound
size up to 45 mm × 30 mm) = £4.50; medium
(wound size up to 110 mm × 75 mm) = £6.50; large
(wound size up to 175 mm × 110 mm) = £8.50;
extra large (horizontal wound up to 245 mm ×
160 mm) = £15.00
Wound pouch, *bung closure*, small (wound size up to
45 mm × 30 mm) = £5.00; medium (wound size up
to 110 mm × 75 mm) = £7.00; large (wound size up
to 175 mm × 110 mm) = £9.50; extra large
(horizontal or vertical wound up to 245 mm ×
160 mm) = £17.00, (vertical incision wound up to
290 mm × 130 mm) = £17.00; (horizontal wound up
to 245 mm × 160 mm), *with access window* = £19.00
Access window, for use with *Eakin*® pouches =
£7.00

Oakmed® Option (OakMed)
Wound Manager, extra small (wound size up to
90 mm × 180 mm) = £11.00; small (horizontal
wound size up to 245 mm × 160 mm) = £12.23;
medium (vertical wound size up to 90 mm ×
260 mm) = £12.50; large (wound size up to 160 mm
× 260 mm) = £14.90; square (vertical wound up to
160 mm × 200 mm) = £13.05
Wound Manager, *with access port*, extra small
(wound size up to 90 mm × 180 mm) = £12.02;
small (horizontal wound size up to 245 mm ×
160 mm) = £12.77; medium (vertical wound size up
to 90 mm × 260 mm) = £13.05; large (wound size
up to 160 mm × 260 mm) = £15.93; square (vertical
wound size up to 160 mm × 200 mm) = £13.59
Wound Manager, *cut-to-fit*, small (10–30 mm) =
£2.25, medium (10–50 mm) = £2.49, large (10–
50 mm) = £2.61

Welland® (CliniMed)
Fistula bag, wound manager, *cut-to-fit* (wound size
up to 40 mm × 70 mm) = £2.54

Wound Drainage Collector (Hollister)
Pouch, drainable, small (wound size up to 76 mm) =
£7.45, medium (wound size up to 95 mm) = £8.13,
large (wound size up to 100 mm × 200 mm) =
£16.10

A5.5.3 Physical debridement pads

DebriSoft® is a pad that is used for the debridement of
superficial wounds containing loose slough and debris,
and for the removal of hyperkeratosis from the skin.
DebriSoft® must be fully moistened with a wound
cleansing solution before use and is not appropriate
for use as a wound dressing.

DebriSoft® (Activa)
Pad, polyester fibres with bound edges and knitted
outer surface coated with polyacrylate, 10 cm ×
10 cm = £6.19

---

1. ⒿⒽⓈ Except in Sterile Dressing Pack with Non-woven
   Pads

A5.6 Complex adjunct therapies

Topical negative pressure (or vacuum-assisted) therapy requires specific wound dressings for use with the vacuum-pump equipment.

Other complex adjunct therapies include sterile larvae (maggots).

A5.6.1 Topical negative pressure therapy

◢Vacuum assisted closure products

Exsu-Fast® (Synergy Healthcare)
Dressing kit, Kit 1 (small wound, low exudate) = £28.04; Kit 2 (large wound, heavy exudate) = £35.83; Kit 3 (large wound, medium to low exudate) = £35.83; Kit 4 (small wound, heavy exudate) = £28.04

Renasys® F/P (S&N Hlth.)
Dressing kit, foam dressing with round drain (plus port, drapes and fixation film), small = £19.49, medium = £22.64, large = £26.85, extra large = £45.28

Renasys® G (S&N Hlth.)
Dressing kit, non-adherent gauze and transparent film dressing, with flat drain, small = £16.64, medium = £20.86, large = £26.48; round drain, small = £16.64, large = £26.48; channel drain, medium = £20.86

V.A.C.® (KCI Medical)
GranuFoam® dressing kit, polyurethane foam dressing (with adhesive drapes and pad connector), 10 cm × 7.5 cm × 3.3 cm (small) = £21.73, 18 cm × 12.5 cm × 3.3 cm (medium) = £25.87, 26 cm × 15 cm × 3.3 cm (large) = £30.01; bridge dressing kit (for diabetic foot wound) = £30.63; *with silver*, small = £31.86, medium = £36.96

Simplace® dressing kit, spiral-cut polyurethane foam dressings, vapour-permeable adhesive film dressings (with adhesive drapes and pad connector), small = £25.43, medium = £29.23

WhiteFoam®, polyvinyl alcohol foam dressing 10 cm × 7.5 cm (small) = £10.18, 10 cm × 15 cm (large) = £16.29; dressing kit (with adhesive drape and pad connector), 10 cm × 7.5 cm (small) = £24.77, 10 cm × 15 cm (large) = £32.06

Venturi® (Talley)
Wound sealing kit, flat drain, standard = £15.00, large = £17.50; channel drain = £15.00

WoundASSIST® (Huntleigh)
Wound pack, small–medium = £20.81, medium–large = £23.85, extra large = £34.05; channel drain, small–medium = £20.81, medium–large = £23.85

◢Wound drainage collection devices

ActiV.A.C.® (KCI Medical)
Canister (with gel), 300 mL = £26.91

Renasys® Go (S&N Hlth.)
Canister kit (with solidifier), 300 mL = £18.77, 750 mL = £25.88

S-Canister® (S&N Hlth.)
Canister kit, 250 mL (with solidifier) = £19.00

V.A.C Freedom® (KCI Medical)
Canister (with gel), 300 mL = £27.58

Venturi® (Talley)
Canister kit, (with solidifier) = £12.50; *Compact* canister kit (with solidifier) = £12.50

V1STA® (S&N Hlth.)
Canister kit, 250 mL (with solidifier) = £19.15, 800 mL (with solidifier) = £21.27

WoundASSIST® (Huntleigh)
Canister, 500 mL = £20.30

◢Accessories

Renasys® (S&N Hlth.)
Port for foam dressing = £9.31, Y-connector = £3.10

V.A.C.® (KCI Medical)
Drape = £8.97. Gel for canister = £3.59. Sensa T.R.A.C. pad = £10.29. T.R.A.C. Y-connector = £2.94

Venturi® (Talley)
Gel patches, adhesive, pack of 5 = £15.00. Y-connector, pack of 5 = £15.00

WoundASSIST® (Huntleigh)
Gel strip = £3.37

A5.7 Wound care accessories

A5.7.1 Dressing packs

The role of dressing packs is very limited. They are used to provide a clean or sterile working surface; some packs shown below include cotton wool balls, which are not recommended for use on wounds.

Multiple Pack Dressing No. 1
(Drug Tariff). Contains absorbent cotton, absorbent cotton gauze type 13 light (sterile), open-wove bandages (banded). 1 pack = £4.09

Non-Drug Tariff Specification Sterile Dressing Pack
Dressit® contains vitrex gloves, large apron, disposable bag, paper towel, softswabs, adsorbent pad, sterile field = 60p (Richardson)
Nurse It® contains latex-free, powder-free nitrile gloves, sterile laminated paper sheet, large apron, non-woven swabs, paper towel, disposable bag, compartmented tray, disposable forceps, paper measuring tape = 52p (Medicare)
Polyfield® Nitrile Patient Pack contains powder-free nitrile gloves, laminate sheet, non-woven swabs, towel, polythene disposable bag, apron = 52p (Shermond)
Propax® SDP contains paper towel, disposable bag, gauze swabs, dressing pad, sterile field = 46p (BSN Medical)
Woundcare® contains nitrile gloves, sterile field, compartmented tray, large apron, disposable bag, non-woven swabs, drape = 44p (Frontier)

Sterile Dressing Pack

(Drug Tariff specification 10). Contains gauze and cotton tissue pad, gauze swabs, absorbent cotton wool balls, absorbent paper towel, water repellent inner wrapper. 1 pack = 51p (Synergy Healthcare—*Vernaid*®)

Sterile Dressing Pack with Non-woven Pads

(Drug Tariff specification 35). Contains non-woven fabric covered dressing pad, non-woven fabric swabs, absorbent cotton wool balls, absorbent paper towel, water repellent inner wrapper. 1 pack = 50p (Synergy Healthcare—*Vernaid*®)

A5.7.2 Woven and fabric swabs

Gauze Swab, BP 1988

Consists of absorbent cotton gauze type 13 light or absorbent cotton and viscose gauze type 1 folded into squares or rectangles of 8-ply with no cut edges exposed, sterile, 7.5 cm × 7.5 cm 5-pad packet = 39p; non-sterile, 10 cm × 10 cm, 100-pad packet = £1.37 (most suppliers)

Filmated Gauze Swab, BP 1988

As for Gauze Swab, but with thin layer of Absorbent Cotton enclosed within, non-sterile, 10 cm × 10 cm, 100-pad packet = £3.67 (Synergy Healthcare—*Cotfil*®)

Non-woven Fabric Swab

(Drug Tariff specification 28). Consists of non-woven fabric folded 4-ply; alternative to gauze swabs, type 13 light, sterile, 7.5 cm × 7.5 cm, 5-pad packet = 25p; non-sterile, 10 cm × 10 cm, 100-pad packet = 79p

Filmated Non-woven Fabric Swab

(Drug Tariff specification 29). Film of viscose fibres enclosed within non-woven viscose fabric folded 8-ply, non-sterile, 10 cm × 10 cm, 100-pad packet = £3.55 (Systagenix—*Regal*®)

A5.7.3 Surgical adhesive tapes

Adhesive tapes are useful for retaining dressings on joints or awkward body parts. These tapes, particularly those containing rubber, can cause irritant and allergic reactions in susceptible patients; synthetic adhesives have been developed to overcome this problem, but they, too, may sometimes be associated with reactions. Synthetic adhesive, or silicon adhesive, tapes can be used for patients with skin reactions to plasters and strapping containing rubber, or undergoing prolonged treatment.

Adhesive tapes that are occlusive may cause skin maceration. Care is needed not to apply these tapes under tension, to avoid creating a tourniquet effect. If applied over joints they need to be orientated so that the area of maximum extensibility of the fabric is in the direction of movement of the limb.

◀ Permeable adhesive tapes

Elastic Adhesive Tape, BP 1988

(Elastic Adhesive Plaster). Woven fabric, elastic in warp (crepe-twisted cotton threads), weft of cotton and/or viscose threads, spread with adhesive mass containing zinc oxide. 4.5 m stretched × 2.5 cm = £1.71 (S&N—*Elastoplast*®)

For 5 cm width, see Elastic Adhesive Bandage

Permeable, Apertured Non-Woven Synthetic Adhesive Tape, BP 1988

Non-woven fabric with a polyacrylate adhesive. Hypafix®, 5 cm × 5 m = £1.36, 10 cm × 5 m = £2.28, 10 m (all): 2.5 cm = £1.58, 5 cm = £2.51, 10 cm = £4.38, 15 cm = £6.49, 20 cm = £8.61, 30 cm = £12.45 (BSN Medical)

Mefix®, 5 m (all): 2.5 cm = 98p, 5 cm = £1.72; 10 cm = £2.76, 15 cm = £3.76, 20 cm = £4.82, 30 cm = £6.91 (Mölnlycke)

Omnifix®, 10 m (all): 5 cm = £2.28, 10 cm = £3.84, 15 cm = £5.66 (Hartmann)

Primafix®, 5 cm × 10 m = £1.50, 10 cm × 10 m = £2.20, 15 cm × 10 m = £3.25, 20 cm × 10 m = £4.00 (S&N Hlth.)

Permeable Non-woven Synthetic Adhesive Tape, BP 1988

Backing of paper-based or non-woven textile material spread with a polymeric adhesive mass:

Clinipore®, 5 m (all) 1.25 cm = 35p, 2.5 cm = 59p, 5 cm = 99p; 2.5 cm × 10 m = 73p (Clinisupplies)

Leukofix®, 5 m (all) 1.25 cm = 52p, 2.5 cm = 84p, 5 cm = £1.47 (BSN Medical)

Leukopor®, 5 m (all) 1.25 cm = 46p, 2.5 cm = 72p, 5 cm = £1.27 (BSN Medical)

Mediplast®, 5 m (all) 1.25 cm = 30p, 2.5 cm = 50p (Neomedic)

Micropore®, 5 m (all) 1.25 cm = 60p, 2.5 cm = 89p, 5 cm = £1.57 (3M)

Scanpor®, 5 m (all) 1.25 cm = 41p, 2.5 cm = 66p, 5 cm = £1.14; 10 m (all), 1.25 cm = 53p, 2.5 cm = 88p, 5 cm = £1.68, 7.5 cm = £2.46 (BioDiagnostics)

Transpore®, 5 m (all) 1.25 cm = 51p, 2.5 cm = 82p, 5 cm = £1.44 (3M)

Where no brand stated by prescriber, net price of tape supplied not to exceed 35p (1.25 cm), 59p (2.5 cm), 99p (5 cm)

Permeable Woven Synthetic Adhesive Tape, BP 1988

Non-extensible closely woven fabric, spread with a polymeric adhesive. 5 m (all): 1.25 cm = 80p, 2.5 cm = £1.17; 5 cm = £2.03 (Beiersdorf—*Leukosilk*®)

Silicone adhesive tape

Soft silicone, water-resistant, knitted fabric, polyurethane film adhesive tape

Insil®, 2 cm × 3 m = £5.60, 4 cm × 1.5 m = £5.60 (Insight)

Mepitac®, 2 cm × 3 m = £6.56, 4 cm × 1.5 m = £6.56 (Mölnlycke)

Siltape®, 2 cm × 3 m = £5.60, 4 cm × 1.5 m = £5.60 (Advancis)

Zinc Oxide Adhesive Tape, BP 1988

(Zinc Oxide Plaster). Fabric, plain weave, warp and weft of cotton and/or viscose, spread with an adhesive containing zinc oxide. 5 m (all): 1.25 cm = 97p; 2.5 cm = £1.40; 5 cm = £2.37; 7.5 cm = £3.57 (most suppliers)

Zinc Oxide Adhesive Tape
Mediplast®, 5 m (all), 1.25 cm = 82p, 2.5 cm =
£1.19, 5 cm = £1.99, 7.5 cm = £2.99 (Neomedic)
Strappal®, 5 m (all): 2.5 cm = £1.30, 5 cm = £2.20,
7.5 cm = £3.31 (BSN Medical)

◢ Occlusive adhesive tapes

Impermeable Plastic Adhesive Tape, BP 1988
Extensible water-impermeable plastic film spread
with an adhesive mass. 2.5 cm × 3 m = £1.36;
2.5 cm × 5 m = £2.03; 5 cm × 5 m = £2.57; 7.5 cm
× 5 m = £3.74 (BSN Medical—Sleek®)

**Impermeable Plastic Synthetic Adhesive Tape, BP
1988**
Extensible water-impermeable plastic film spread
with a polymeric adhesive mass. 5 m (both): 2.5 cm
= £1.72; 5 cm = £3.27 (3M—Blenderm®)

A5.7.4 Adhesive dressings

Adhesive dressings (also termed 'island dressings') have
a limited role for minor wounds only. The inclusion of
an antiseptic is not particularly useful and may cause
skin irritation in susceptible subjects.

◢ Vapour permeable adhesive dressings

**Vapour-permeable Waterproof Plastic Wound
Dressing, BP 1993**
(former Drug Tariff title: Semipermeable Waterproof
Plastic Wound Dressing). Consists of absorbent pad,
may be dyed and impregnated with suitable
antiseptic (see under Elastic Adhesive Dressing),
attached to piece of semi-permeable waterproof
surgical adhesive tape, to leave suitable adhesive
margin; both pad and margin covered with suitable
protector (S&N Hlth—Elastoplast Airstrip®)

A5.7.5 Skin closure dressings

Skin closure strips are used as an alternative to sutures
for minor cuts and lacerations. Skin tissue adhesive
(BNF section 13.10.5) can be used for closure of
minor skin wounds and for additional suture support.

Skin closure strips, sterile
Leukostrip®, 6.4 mm × 76 mm, 3 strips per
envelope. 10 envelopes = £5.95 (S&N Hlth.)
Omnistrip®, 6 mm × 76 mm, 3 strips per envelope.
50 envelopes = £22.89 (Hartmann)
Steri-strip®, 6 mm × 75 mm, 3 strips per envelope.
12 envelopes = £8.52 (3M)
Drug Tariff specifies that these are specifically for personal
administration by the prescriber

A5.8 Bandages

According to their structure and performance bandages
are used for dressing retention, for support, and for
compression.

A5.8.1 Non-extensible bandages

Bandages made from non-extensible, woven fabrics
have generally been replaced by more conformable
products, therefore their role is now extremely limited.
Triangular calico bandage has a role as a sling.

Open-wove Bandage, Type 1 BP 1988
Cotton cloth, plain weave, warp of cotton, weft of
cotton, viscose, or combination, one continuous
length. 5 m (all): 2.5 cm = 31p; 5 cm = 53p; 7.5 cm =
75p; 10 cm = 98p (most suppliers)

Triangular Calico Bandage, BP 1980
Unbleached calico right-angled triangle, 90 cm ×
90 cm × 1.27 m = £1.17 (most suppliers)

A5.8.2 Light-weight conforming bandages

Lightweight conforming bandages are used for dressing
retention, with the aim of keeping the dressing close to
the wound without inhibiting movement or restricting
blood flow. The elasticity of **conforming-stretch bandages** (also termed contour bandages) is greater than
that of **cotton conforming bandages.**

Conforming Bandage (Synthetic)
Fabric, plain weave, warp of polyamide, weft of
viscose. 4 m stretched (all):
Hospiform®, 6 cm = 13p, 8 cm = 16p, 10 cm = 18p,
12 cm = 22p (Hartmann)

Cotton Conforming Bandage, BP 1988
Cotton fabric, plain weave, treated to impart some
elasticity to warp and weft. 3.5 m (all): type A, 5 cm
= 64p, 7.5 cm = 78p, 10 cm = 97p, 15 cm = £1.32
(BSN Medical—Easifix Crinx®)

**Knitted Polyamide and Cellulose Contour
Bandage, BP 1988**
Fabric, knitted warp of polyamide filament, weft of
cotton or viscose, fast edges, one continuous length.
4 m stretched (all):
Easifix K®, 2.5 cm = 9p, 5 cm = 10p, 7.5 cm = 15p,
10 cm = 17p, 15 cm = 30p (BSN Medical)
K-Band®, 5 cm = 19p, 7 cm = 24p, 10 cm = 27p,
15 cm = 47p (Urgo)
Knit-Band®, 5 cm = 10p, 7 cm = 15p, 10 cm = 17p,
15 cm = 30p (CliniMed)
Knit Fix®, 5 cm = 12p, 7 cm = 17p, 10 cm = 17p,
15 cm = 30p (Steraid)

Polyamide and Cellulose Contour Bandage
Peha-haft®, cohesive, latex-free, 4 m (all) 2.5 cm =
69p, 4 cm = 45p, 6 cm = 53p, 8 cm = 63p, 10 cm =
72p, 12 cm = 85p (Hartmann)
PremierBand®, 4 m (all); 5 cm = 12p, 7.5 cm = 14p,
10 cm = 17p, 15 cm = 25p (Shermond)

**Polyamide and Cellulose Contour Bandage, BP
1988**
(Nylon and Viscose Stretch Bandage)
Fabric, plain weave, warp of polyamide filament, weft
of cotton or viscose, fast edges, one continuous
length, 4 m stretched (all):
Acti-Wrap®, cohesive, latex-free, 6 cm = 44p, 8 cm =
64p, 10 cm = 76p (Activa)
Easifix®, 2.5 cm = 9p, 5 cm = 33p, 7.5 cm = 40p,
10 cm = 48p, 15 cm = 81p (BSN Medical)

Kontour®, cohesive, 5 cm = 28p, 7.5 cm = 35p, 10 cm = 40p, 15 cm = 66p (Easigrip)
Mollelast®, latex-free, 4 cm = 28p (Activa)
Slinky®, 7.5 cm = 57p, 10 cm = 68p, 15 cm = 98p (Mölnlycke)
Stayform®, 5 cm = 29p, 7.5 cm = 36p, 10 cm = 40p, 15 cm = 68p (Robinsons)

A5.8.3 Tubular bandages and garments

Tubular bandages are available in different forms, according to the function required of them. Some are used under orthopaedic casts and some are suitable for protecting areas to which creams or ointments (other than those containing potent corticosteroids) have been applied. The conformability of the elasticated versions makes them particularly suitable for retaining dressings on difficult parts of the body or for soft tissue injury, but their use as the only means of applying pressure to an oedematous limb or to a varicose ulcer is not appropriate, since the pressure they exert is inadequate.

Compression hosiery (section A5.9.1) reduces the recurrence of venous leg ulcers and should be considered for use after wound healing.

Silk clothing is available as an alternative to elasticated viscose stockinette garments, for use in the management of severe eczema and allergic skin conditions (see below).

◀ **Elasticated**

Elasticated Surgical Tubular Stockinette, Foam padded

(Drug Tariff specification 25). Fabric as for Elasticated Tubular Bandage with polyurethane foam lining. Heel, elbow, knee, small = £2.86, medium = £3.09, large = £3.30; sacral, medium, and large (all) = £14.76 (Medlock—*Tubipad®*)
Uses   relief of pressure and elimination of friction in relevant area; porosity of foam lining allows normal water loss from skin surface

Elasticated Tubular Bandage, BP 1993

(formerly Elasticated Surgical Tubular Stockinette). Knitted fabric, elasticated threads of rubber-cored polyamide or polyester with cotton or cotton and viscose yarn, tubular. Lengths 50 cm and 1 m, widths 6.25 cm, 6.75 cm, 7.5 cm, 8.75 cm, 10 cm, 12 cm; Synergy—*Comfigrip®*; Easigrip—*EasiGRIP®*; Sallis—*Eesiban®*; Medlock—*Tubigrip®*. Where no size stated by prescriber the 50 cm length should be supplied and width endorsed

Elasticated Viscose Stockinette

(Drug Tariff specification 46). Lightweight plain-knitted elasticated tubular bandage.
Acti-Fast®, 3.5 cm red line (small limb), length 1 m = 62p; 5 cm green line (medium limb), length 1 m = 65p, 3 m = £1.90, 5 m = £3.30; 7.5 cm blue line (large limb), length 1 m = 90p, 3 m = £2.50, 5 m = £4.40; 10.75 cm yellow line (child trunk), length 1 m = £1.45, 3 m = £4.10, 5 m = £7.10; 17.5 cm beige line (adult trunk), length 1 m = £2.15; 20 cm purple line (large adult trunk), length 1 m = £3.20, 5 m = £16.15 (Activa)
CliniFast®, 3.5 cm red line (small limb), length 1 m = 56p; 5 cm green line (medium limb), length 1 m = 58p, 3 m = £1.62, 5 m = £2.81; 7.5 cm blue line

(large limb), length 1 m = 77p, 3 m = £2.13, 5 m = £3.74; 10.75 cm yellow line (child trunk), length 1 m = £1.20, 3 m = £3.49, 5 m = £6.04; 17.5 cm beige line (adult trunk), length 1 m = £1.83; *vest (long-sleeved)*, 6–24 months = £7.13, 2–5 years = £9.50, 5–8 years = £10.69, 8–11 years = £11.88, 11–14 years = £11.88, adult, small, = £12.75, medium = £14.54, large = £16.58; *vest (short-sleeved)*, adult, small = £12.50, medium = £14.25, large = £16.25; *tights (pair)* 6–24 months = £7.13; *leggings (pair)* 2–5 years = £9.50, 5–8 years = £10.69, 8–11 years = £11.88, 11–14 years = £11.88, adult, small, = £12.75, medium = £14.54, large = £16.58; *cycle shorts*, adult, small = £12.50, medium = £14.25, large = £16.25; *socks (pair)* up to 8 years = £2.97, 8–14 years = £2.97; *mittens (pair)* up to 24 months = £2.97, 2–8 years = £2.97, 8–14 years = £2.97; *gloves*, child, small, medium, large = £4.99, adult, small, medium, large = £4.99; *clava*, 6 months–5 years = £5.85, 5–14 years = £6.75 (Clinisupplies)
Comfifast®, 3.5 cm red line (small limb), length 1 m = 56p; 5 cm green line (medium limb), length 1 m = 58p, 3 m = £1.62, 5 m = £2.81; 7.5 cm blue line (large limb), length 1 m = 77p, 3 m = £2.13, 5 m = £3.74; 10.75 cm yellow line (child trunk), length 1 m = £1.20, 3 m = £3.49, 5 m = £6.04; 17.5 cm beige line (adult trunk), length 1 m = £1.83 (Synergy)
Comfifast® Easy Wrap, *vest (long-sleeved)*, 6–24 months = £7.13, 2–5 years = £9.50, 5–8 years = £10.69, 8–11 years = £11.88, 11–14 years = £11.88, adult, small = £12.75, medium = £14.54, large = £16.58; *tights (pair)*, 6–24 months = £7.13; *leggings (pair)*, 2–5 years = £9.50, 5–8 years = £10.69, 8–11 years = £11.88, 11–14 years = £11.88, adult, small = £12.75, medium = £14.54, large = £16.58; *socks (pair)*, up to 8 years = £2.97, 8–14 = £2.97; *mittens (pair)*, up to 24 months = £2.97, 2–8 years = £2.97, 8–14 years = £2.97; *clava*, 6 months–5 years = £5.85, 5–14 years = £6.75 (Synergy)
Comfifast® Multistretch, 3.5 cm red line (small limb), length 1 m = 72p; 5 cm green line (medium limb), length 1 m = 78p, 3 m = £2.23, 5 m = £3.82; 7.5 cm blue line (large limb), length 1 m = £1.05, 3 m = £2.93, 5 m = £5.12; 10.75 cm yellow line (child trunk), length 1 m = £1.67, 3 m = £4.78, 5 m = £8.21; 17.5 cm beige line (adult trunk), length 1 m = £2.49 (Synergy Healthcare)
Coverflex®, 3.5 cm red line (small limb), length 1 m = 78p; 5 cm green line (medium limb), length 1 m = 81p, 3 m = £2.38, 5 m = £4.10; 7.5 cm blue line (large limb), length 1 m = £1.13, 3 m = £2.70, 5 m = £5.35; 10.75 cm yellow line (child trunk), length 1 m = £1.78, 3 m = £5.13, 5 m = £9.02; 17.5 cm beige line (adult trunk), length 1 m = £2.38 (Hartmann)
Easifast®, 3.5 cm red line (small limb), length 1 m = 65p; 5 cm green line (medium limb), length 1 m = 69p, 3 m = £1.95, 5 m = £3.40; 7.5 cm blue line (large limb), length 1 m = 94p, 3 m = £2.60, 5 m = £4.50; 10.75 cm yellow line (child trunk), length 1 m = £1.50, 3 m = £4.25, 5 m = £7.20; 17.5 cm beige line (adult trunk), length 1 m = £1.90 (Easigrip)
Skinnies®, *body-suit*, premature, 0–3 months, or 3–6 months = £15.90, 6–24 months = £17.90; *clava*, 6 months–5 years = £6.62, 5–14 years = £7.60; *gloves* child (small) = £5.20, (medium or large) = £5.25, adult (small) = £5.20, (medium or large) = £5.25; *leggings (pair)*, 6–24 months = £10.30, 2–5 years = £13.50, 5–8 years = £15.25, 8–11 years or 11–14 years = £16.90, adult (small) = £20.90, (medium) =

£22.80, (large) = £24.70; *mittens*, 0–24 months, 2–8 years, or 8–14 years = £3.80; *socks, ankle (pair)*, 6 months–8 years or 8–14 years = £4.20; *socks, knee (pair)*, child (small, medium, or large, up to shoe size 4) = £13.70, adult (shoe size 4–6, 6–8, 8–11, or size 11+) = £13.70; *vest (long-sleeved)*, 6–24 months = £10.30, 2–5 years = £13.50, 5–8 years = £15.25, 8–11 years or 11–14 years = £16.90, adult (small) = £20.90, (medium) = £22.80, (large) = £24.70; *vest (short-sleeved)*, 6–24 months = £10.20, 2–5 years = £13.40, 5–8 years = £15.10, 8–11 years or 11–14 years = £16.80, adult (small) = £20.80, (medium) = £22.70, (large) = £24.60; *vest (sleeveless)*, 6–24 months = £10.20, 2–5 years = £13.40, 5–8 years = £15.15, 8–11 years = £16.80, 11–14 years = £16.80, adult (small) = £20.80, (medium) = £22.70, (large) = £24.60 (Skinnies)

Tubifast® 2-way stretch, 3.5 cm red line (small limb), length 1 m = 88p; 5 cm green line (medium limb), length 1 m = 95p, 3 m = £2.70, 5 m = £4.61; 7.5 cm blue line (large limb), length 1 m = £1.26, 3 m = £3.55, 5 m = £6.19; 10.75 cm yellow line (child trunk), length 1 m = £2.02, 3 m = £5.78, 5 m = £9.92; 20 cm purple line (large adult trunk), length 1 m = £3.27, 5 m = £16.00; *vest (long-sleeved)*, 6–24 months = £10.97, 2–5 years = £14.63, 5–8 years = £16.46, 8–11 years = £18.28, 11–14 years = £18.28; *tights (pair)*, 6–24 months = £10.97; *leggings (pair)*, 2–5 years = £14.63, 5–8 years = £16.46, 8–11 years = £18.28, 11–14 years = £18.28; *socks (pair)*, one-size = £4.58; *gloves*, (small-medium or medium-large adult, extra small or small child) = £5.50 (Mölnlycke)

◀ Non-elasticated

Cotton Stockinette, Bleached, BP 1988

Knitted fabric, cotton yarn, tubular length, 1 m (all), 2.5 cm = 37p; 5 cm = 58p; 7.5 cm = 69p; 6 m × 10 cm = £4.75 (Sallis—Eesiban®)

Uses   1 m lengths, basis (with wadding) for Plaster of Paris bandages etc.; 6 m length, compression bandage

Ribbed Cotton and Viscose Surgical Tubular Stockinette, BP 1988

Knitted fabric of 1:1 ribbed structure, singles yarn spun from blend of two-thirds cotton and one-third viscose fibres, tubular. Length 5 m (all):

Type A (lightweight): arm/leg (child), arm (adult) 5 cm = £2.45; arm (OS adult), leg (adult) 7.5 cm = £3.22; leg (OS adult) 10 cm = £4.27; trunk (child) 15 cm = £6.15; trunk (adult) 20 cm = £7.11; trunk (OS adult) 25 cm = £8.50 (Mölnlycke)

Type B (heavyweight): sizes as for Type A, net price £2.55–£8.83 (Sallis—Eesiban®)

Drug Tariff specifies various combinations of sizes to provide sufficient material for part or full body coverage

Uses   protective dressings with tar-based and other non-steroid ointments

◀ Silk Clothing

Knitted, medical grade silk clothing can be used as an adjunct to normal treatment for severe eczema and allergic skin conditions. When used in combination with medical creams and ointments, care should be taken to ensure that the medication is fully absorbed into the skin before the silk clothing is worn; silk garments are not suitable for use in direct contact with emollients used in 'wet wrapping techniques'.

DermaSilk® (Espere)

Knitted silk fabric, hypoallergenic, sericin-free, *body suit*, child 0–3 months (height 62 cm) = £36.18, 3–6 months (height 68 cm) = £36.82, 6–9 months (height 74 cm) = £37.87, 9–12 months (height 74 cm) = 38.25, 12–18 months (height 86 cm) = £38.92, 18–24 months (height 92 cm) = £39.29, 2–3 years (height 98 cm) = £38.71, 3–4 years (height 110 cm) = £41.03; *boxer shorts*, adult (male), small–XXXL = £39.95; *briefs*, 3–4 years = £20.95, 5–6 years = £20.95, 7–8 years = £20.95, 10–12 years = £20.95, adult (female), small–XXL = £29.39; *facial mask*, child (head circumference up to 47 cm) = £15.80, child (head circumference up to 50 cm) = £15.80, teen or adult = £20.19; *gloves*, adult (small, medium, large, or extra large) = £19.96, child (small or medium) = £14.22; *leggings*, child 0–3 months (height 62 cm) = £25.83, 3–6 months (height 68 cm) = £26.28, 6–9 months (height 74 cm) = £27.34, 9–12 months (height 74 cm) = £27.90, 12–18 months (height 86 cm) = £28.39, 18–24 months (height 92 cm) = £28.94, 2–3 years (height 98 cm) = £28.51, 3–4 years (height 110 cm) = £30.50, adult (male), small–XXL = £75.60, adult (female), small–XXL = £75.60; *pyjamas*, child 3–4 years (height 110 cm) = £68.42, 5–6 years (height 120 cm) = £72.63, 7–8 years (height 135 cm) = £75.79, 10–12 years (height 150 cm) = £78.95; *shirt*, roll-neck, 3–4 years = £45.56, 5–6 years = £48.49, 7–8 years = £50.51, 10–12 years = £52.54, adult, small–XXL = £74.72; *shirt*, round-neck, adult (male), small–XXL = £74.72, adult (female), small–XXL = £74.72; *sleeves (tubular)*, length 33 cm = £26.28, 50 cm = £32.50; *undersocks, (heel-less)*, 2 pairs standard or longer length = £23.39; *undersocks*, adult shoe-size 5½–6½, 7–8½, 9–10½, 11–13, child shoe-size 3–8, 9–1, 2–5, 2 pairs = £17.78

DreamSkin® (Dreamskin)

Knitted silk fabric, hypoallergenic, sericin-free, with methyacrylate copolymer and zinc-based antibacterial, *body suit (with foldaway mitts)*, child 0–3 months = £35.15, 0–6 months = £35.65, 3–6 months = £35.65, 6–9 months = £36.67, 9–12 months = £37.20, 12–18 months = £37.69, 18–24 months = £38.20, 2–3 years = £38.71, 3–4 years = £39.73; *briefs or fitted boxers*, 3–4 years = £20.95, 5–6 years = £20.95, 7–8 years = £20.95, 9–10 years = £20.95, 11–12 years = £20.95, adult (male) small–XXL = £32.95, adult (female) small–XXL = £30.95; *eye mask*, one size = £9.95; *gloves*, child (small or medium) = £13.98, adult (small, medium, large, or extra large) = £19.62; *head mask*, child up to 1 year (head circumference 39–45cm) = £15.30, child 1–8 years (head circumference 48–50cm) = £15.30, child 12–18 years = £19.96, adult = £19.96; *baby leggings (with foldaway feet)*, child 0–3 months = £24.95, 0–6 months = £25.45, 3–6 months = £25.45, 6–9 months = £26.47, 9–12 months = £26.98, 12–18 months = £27.49, 18–24 months = £28.00, 2–3 years = £28.51, 3–4 years = £29.53; *leggings (without feet; male or female styles)*, 3–4 years = £29.53, 5–6 years = £30.99, 7–8 years = £31.49, 9–10 years = £31.99, 11–12 years = £32.49, adult small–XXL = £74.74; *pyjamas (male or female styles)*, 3–4 years = £66.25, 5–6 years = £70.33, 7–8 years = £73.39, 9–10 years = £74.95, 11–12 years = £76.45; *shirt*, polo-neck, long-sleeved (male or female styles), 3–4 years = £44.94, 5–6 years = £47.94, 7–8 years = £49.94, 9–10 years = £50.94, 11–12 years = £51.94, adult small–XXL = £73.87; *shirt, round-neck, long-sleeved (male or female styles)*, 3–4 years = £44.95, 5–6 years = £46.95, 7–8 years = £48.95, 9–10 years = £49.95, 11–12 years = £50.95, adult small–XXL = £73.87; *sleeves, (tubular)*, pair, length 33 cm = £25.83, 50 cm = £32.13; *tights*, adult (female) small–XL = £22.95; *undersocks, (liner socks)*, 2 pairs, child shoe-size 3–5½, 6–8½, 9–12, 12½–3½, 4–5½, = £17.58, adult (male) shoe-size 6–8½, 9–11 = £17.58, adult (female) shoe-size 4–5½, 6–8½ = £17.58; *undersocks (heel-less)*, one size = £23.12

A5.8.4 Support bandages

Light support bandages, which include the various forms of crepe bandage, are used in the prevention of oedema; they are also used to provide support for mild sprains and joints but their effectiveness has not been proven for this purpose. Since they have limited extensibility, they are able to provide light support without exerting undue pressure. For a warning against injudicious compression see section A5.8.7.

Crepe Bandage, BP 1988
Fabric, plain weave, warp of wool threads and crepe-twisted cotton threads, weft of cotton threads; stretch bandage. 4.5 m stretched (all): 5 cm = 93p; 7.5 cm = £1.31; 10 cm = £1.71; 15 cm = £2.48 (most suppliers)

Cotton Crepe Bandage
Light support bandage, 4.5 m stretched (all): 5 cm = 48p; 7.5 cm = 67p; 10 cm = 87p; 15 cm = £1.27 (Steraid—*Hospicrepe*® 239)

Cotton Crepe Bandage, BP 1988
Fabric, plain weave, warp of crepe-twisted cotton threads, weft of cotton and/or viscose threads; stretch bandage. 4.5 m stretched (both): 7.5 cm = £2.93; 10 cm = £3.76 (most suppliers)

Cotton, Polyamide and Elastane Bandage
Fabric, cotton, polyamide, and elastane; light support bandage (Type 2), 4.5 m stretched (all)
Hospilite®, 5 cm = 35p, 7.5 cm = 48p, 10 cm = 58p, 15 cm = 85p (Hartmann)
Neosport®, 5 cm = 54p, 7.5 cm = 73p, 10 cm = 91p, 15 cm = £1.12 (Neomedic)
Profore® #2, 10 cm = £1.27, latex-free = £1.35 (S&N Hlth)
Setocrepe®, 10 cm = £1.13 (Mölnlycke)
Soffcrepe®, 5 cm = 65p, 7.5 cm = 92p, 10 cm = £1.16, 15 cm = £1.69 (BSN Medical)

Cotton Stretch Bandage, BP 1988
Fabric, plain weave, warp of crepe-twisted cotton threads, weft of cotton threads; stretch bandage, lighter than cotton crepe, 4.5 m stretched (all):
Hospicrepe® 233, 5 cm = 52p; 7.5 cm = 72p; 10 cm = 96p; 15 cm = £1.36 (Steraid)
PremierBand®, 5 cm = 45p, 7.5 cm = 63p, 10 cm = 79p, 15 cm = £1.18 (Shermond)

Cotton Suspensory Bandage
(Drug Tariff). Type 1: cotton net bag with draw tapes and webbing waistband; small, medium, and large (all) = £1.62, extra large = £1.71. Type 2: cotton net bag with elastic edge and webbing waistband; small = £1.79, medium = £1.84, large = £1.91, extra large = £1.98. Type 3: cotton net bag with elastic edge and webbing waistband with

elastic insertion; small, medium, and large (all) = £1.93; extra large = £2.00. Type supplied to be endorsed

Knitted Elastomer and Viscose Bandage
Knitted fabric, viscose and elastomer yarn.
Type 2 (light support bandage)
CliniLite®, 4.5 m (all), 5 cm = 44p, 7.5 cm = 61p, 10 cm = 80p, 15 cm = £1.16 (Clinisupplies)
K-Lite®, 4.5 m stretched, 5 cm = 52p, 7 cm = 73p, 10 cm = 95p, 15 cm = £1.38; 5.2 m stretched, 10 cm = £1.09 (Urgo)
Knit-Firm®, 4.5 m stretched, 5 cm = 36p, 7 cm = 51p, 10 cm = 66p, 15 cm = 96p (Steraid)
Type 3a (light compression bandage):
CliniPlus®, 8.7 m × 10 cm = £1.80 (Clinisupplies)
Elset®, 6 m stretched, 10 cm = £2.46, 15 cm = £2.66; 8 m stretched, 10 cm = £3.14; 12 m stretched, 15 cm = £5.27 (Mölnlycke)
K-Plus®, 8.7 m stretched, 10 cm = £2.14; long, 10.25 m stretched, 10 cm = £2.47 (Urgo)
Profore® #3, 8.7 m stretched, 10 cm = £3.70, latex-free = £4.02 (S&N Hlth.)
L3, 8.6 m stretched, 10 cm = £2.07 (S&N Hlth.)

A5.8.5 Adhesive bandages

Elastic adhesive bandages are used to provide compression in the treatment of varicose veins and for the support of injured joints; they should no longer be used for the support of fractured ribs and clavicles. They have also been used with **zinc paste bandage** in the treatment of venous ulcers, but they can cause skin reactions in susceptible patients and may not produce sufficient pressures for healing (significantly lower than those provided by other compression bandages).

Elastic Adhesive Bandage, BP 1993
Woven fabric, elastic in warp (crepe-twisted cotton threads), weft of cotton and/or viscose threads spread with adhesive mass containing zinc oxide. 4.5 m stretched (all): 5 cm = £3.45; 7.5 cm = £4.99; 10 cm = £6.64 (BSN Medical—*Elastoplast*® Bandage).
Drug Tariff specifies 7.5 cm width supplied when size not stated

A5.8.6 Cohesive bandages

Cohesive bandages adhere to themselves, but not to the skin, and are useful for providing support for sports use where ordinary stretch bandages might become displaced and adhesive bandages are inappropriate. Care is needed in their application, however, since the loss of ability for movement between turns of the bandage to equalise local areas of high tension carries the potential for creating a tourniquet effect. Cohesive bandages can be used to support sprained joints and as an outer layer for multi-layer compression bandaging; they should not be used if arterial disease is suspected.

◀ Cohesive extensible bandages

Coban® (3M)
Bandage, 6 m (stretched), 10 cm = £2.79

K-Press® (Urgo)
Bandage, 6.5 m × 10 cm (0, short) = £2.78; 7.5 m, 18–25 cm ankle circumference, 8 cm = £3.06, 10 cm = £3.25, 12 cm = £4.09; 10.5 m, 25–32 cm ankle circumference, 8 cm = £3.33, 10 cm = £3.55, 12 cm = £4.48

Profore® #4 (S&N Hlth.)
Bandage, 2.5 m (unstretched) = £3.06, latex-free = £3.32

Ultra Fast® (Robinsons)
Bandage, 6.3 m (stretched), 10 cm = £2.59

A5.8.7   Compression bandages

High compression products are used to provide the high compression needed for the management of gross varices, post-thrombotic venous insufficiency, venous leg ulcers, and gross oedema in average-sized limbs. Their use calls for an expert knowledge of the elastic properties of the products and experience in the technique of providing careful graduated compression. Incorrect application can lead to uneven and inadequate pressures or to hazardous levels of pressure. In particular, injudicious use of compression in limbs with arterial disease has been reported to cause severe skin and tissue necrosis (in some instances calling for amputation). Doppler testing is required before treatment with compression. Oral pentoxifylline (BNF section 2.6.4) can be used as adjunct therapy if a chronic venous leg ulcer does not respond to compression bandaging [unlicensed indication].

◢High compression bandages

PEC High Compression Bandage
Polyamide, elastane, and cotton compression (high) extensible bandage, 3.5 m unstretched, 10 cm = £3.34 (Mölnlycke—*Setopress®*)

VEC High Compression Bandage
Viscose, elastane, and cotton compression (high) extensible bandage, 3 m unstretched (both); 7.5 cm = £2.56; 10 cm = £3.29 (S&N—*Tensopress®*)

High Compression Bandage
Cotton, viscose, nylon, and Lycra® extensible bandage, 3 m (unstretched), 10 cm = £3.42 (ConvaTec— *SurePress®*); 3 m (unstretched), 10 cm = £2.66 (Urgo—*K-ThreeC®*)

◢Short stretch compression bandage

Short stretch bandages help to reduce oedema and promote healing of venous leg ulcers. They are also used to reduce swelling associated with lymphoedema. They are applied at full stretch over padding (*see* Sub-compression Wadding Bandage below) which protects areas of high pressure and sites at high risk of pressure damage.

Actico® (Activa)
Bandage, cohesive, 6 m (all), 4 cm = £2.25, 6 cm = £2.64, 8 cm = £3.03, 10 cm = £3.15, 12 cm = £4.02

Comprilan® (BSN Medical)
Bandage, 5 m (all), 6 cm = £2.55; 8 cm = £2.99; 10 cm = £3.22; 12 cm = £3.92

Rosidal K® (Activa)
Bandage, 5 m (all), 4cm = £1.79, 6cm = £2.50, 8 cm = £2.98, 10 cm = £3.26, 12 cm = £3.95; 10m x 10cm = £5.67

Silkolan® (Urgo)
Bandage, 5 m (all), 8 cm = £3.00; 10 cm = £3.39

◢Sub-compression wadding bandage

Advasoft® (Advancis)
Padding, 3.5 m unstretched, 10 cm = 37p

Cellona® Undercast Padding (Activa)
Padding, 2.75 m unstretched (all): 5 cm = 29p, 7.5 cm = 36p; 10 cm = 44p; 15 cm = 57p

Coban® 2 Comfort Layer (3M)
Padding, 2.7 m unstretched, 10 cm = £5.50

Flexi-Ban® (Activa)
Padding, 3.5 m unstretched, 10cm = 47p

K-Soft® (Urgo)
Padding, absorbent, 3.5 m unstretched, 10 cm = 43p; 4.5 m unstretched, 10 cm = 53p

K-Tech® (Urgo)
Padding, 5 m × 10 cm (0, short) = £3.76; 6 m, 18–25 cm ankle circumference, 8 cm = £4.26, 10 cm = £4.51, 12 cm = £5.69; 7.3 m, 25–32 cm ankle circumference, 8 cm = £4.64, 10 cm = £4.92, 12 cm = £6.21
Note *K-Tech®* also includes a short stretch compressive fabric component

K-Tech® Reduced (Urgo)
Padding, 6 m x 10 cm, 18–25 cm ankle circumference = £4.51; 7.3 m x 10 cm, 25–32 cm ankle circumference = £4.92
Note *K-Tech® Reduced* also includes a short stretch compressive fabric component

Ortho-Band Plus® (Steraid)
Padding, 10 cm × 3.5 cm unstretched = 37p

Profore® #1 (S&N Hlth.)
Padding, viscose fleece, 3.5 m unstretched, 10 cm = 66p, latex-free = 72p

Softexe® (Mölnlycke)
Padding, absorbent, 3.5 m unstretched, 10 cm = 60p

SurePress® (ConvaTec)
Padding, absorbent, 3 m unstretched, 10 cm = 56p

Ultra Soft® (Robinsons)
Padding, absorbent, 3.5 m unstretched, 10 cm = 39p

Velband® (BSN Medical)
Padding, absorbent, 4.5 m unstretched, 10 cm = 68p

A5.8.8   Multi-layer compression bandaging

Multi-layer compression bandaging systems are an alternative to High Compression Bandages (section A5.8.7) for the treatment of venous leg ulcers. Compression is achieved by the combined effects of two or three extensible bandages applied over a layer of orthopaedic wadding and a wound contact dressing.

◢ **Four layer systems**

K-Four® (Urgo)
K-Four® # 1 (*K-Soft®*—see Sub-compression Wadding Bandage, p. 59); *K-Four®* # 2 (*K-Lite®*—see Knitted Elastomer and Viscose Bandage, p. 58); *K-Four®* # 3 (*K-Plus®*—see Knitted Elastomer and Viscose Bandage, p. 58); *K-Three C®*—see High compression bandages, p. 59; *K-Four®* # 4 (*Ko-Flex®*), 6 m (stretched), 10 cm = £2.84; 7 m (stretched), 10 cm = £3.25

Multi-layer compression bandaging kit, four layer system, for ankle circumference up to 18 cm = £6.73, 18–25 cm = £6.44, 25–30 cm = £6.44, above 30 cm = £8.87; *reduced compression*, 18 cm and above = £4.21

Profore® (S&N Hlth.)
Profore® wound contact layer (see Knitted Viscose Primary Dressing, p. 37); *Profore®* #1 (see Sub-compression Wadding Bandage, p. 59); *Profore®* #2 (see Cotton, Polyamide and Elastane Bandage, p. 58); *Profore®* #3 (see Knitted Elastomer and Viscose Bandage, p. 58); *Profore®* #4 (see Cohesive bandages, p. 59); *Profore®* Plus 3 m (unstretched), 10 cm = £3.46, latex-free = £3.70

Multi-layer compression bandaging kit, four layer system, for ankle circumference up to 18 cm = £9.58, 18–25 cm = £8.92, 25–30 cm = £7.41, above 30 cm = £11.09, latex-free, 18–25 cm = £9.53; *Profore Lite®* above 18 cm = £5.15, latex-free = £5.60

System 4® (Mölnlycke)
System 4® #1 (*Softexe®*—see Sub-compression Wadding Bandage, p. 59); *System 4®* #2 (*Setocrepe®*—see Cotton, Polyamide and Elastane Bandage, p. 58); *System 4®* #3 (*Elset®*—see Knitted Elastomer and Viscose Bandage, p. 58); *System 4®* #4 (*Meban®*)

Multi-layer compression bandaging kit, four layer system, for ankle circumference 18–25 cm = £7.46

Ultra Four® (Robinsons)
Ultra Four® #1 (*Ultra Soft®*—see Sub-compression Wadding Bandage, p. 59); *Ultra Four®* #2 (*Ultra Lite®*) 10 cm × 4.5 cm (stretched) = 85p; *Ultra Four®* #3 (*Ultra Plus®*) 10 cm × 8.7 cm (stretched) = £1.89; *Ultra Four®* #4 (*Ultra Fast®*—see Cohesive Bandages, p. 59)

Multi-layer compression bandaging kit, four layer system, for ankle circumference up to 18 cm = £6.41, 18–25 cm = £5.67; *Ultra Four®* RC (reduced compression) 18–25 cm = £4.14

◢ **Two layer systems**

Coban® 2 (3M)
Multi-layer compression bandaging kit, two layer system (latex-free, foam bandage and cohesive compression bandage), one size = £8.08; *Coban® 2 Lite* (reduced compression), one size = £8.08

K-Two® (Urgo)
K-Tech® (see Sub-compression Wadding Bandages, p. 59); *K-Press®* (see Cohesive bandages, p. 59)
Multi-layer compression bandaging kit, two layer system, size 0 (short) = £6.55; 18–25 cm ankle circumference, 8 cm = £7.32, 10 cm = £7.76, 12 cm = £9.78; 25–32 cm ankle circumference, 8 cm = £7.96, 10 cm = £8.48, 12 cm = £10.69

K-Two® Latex Free, *K-Tech®* (see Sub-compression Wadding Bandages, above); *K-Press®* Latex Free

Multi-layer compression bandaging kit, two layer system, for ankle circumference 18–25 cm = £8.38; 25–32 cm = £9.16

K-Two® Reduced, *K-Tech®* Reduced (see Sub-compression Wadding Bandages, above); *K-Press®* (see Cohesive Bandages, p. 59)

Multi-layer compression bandaging kit, two layer system, for ankle circumference 18–25 cm = £7.76; 25–32 cm = £8.48

K-Two® Reduced Latex Free, *K-Tech®* (see Sub-compression Wadding Bandages, above); *K-Press®* Reduced Latex Free

Multi-layer compression bandaging kit, two layer system, for ankle circumference 18–25 cm = £8.38; 25–32 cm = £9.16

K-Two® Start, *UrgoStart®* Contact (see Protease-modulating matrix, p. 51); *K-Tech®* (see Sub-compression Wadding Bandages, p. 59); *K-Press®* (see Cohesive Bandages, p. 59)

Multi-layer compression bandaging kit, two-layer system, for ankle circumference 18–25cm = £9.68; 25–32cm = £10.33

A5.8.9   Medicated bandages

Zinc Paste Bandage has been used with compression bandaging for the treatment of venous leg ulcers. However, paste bandages are associated with hypersensitivity reactions and should be used with caution.

Zinc paste bandages are also used with **coal tar** or **ichthammol** in chronic lichenified skin conditions such as chronic eczema (ichthammol often being preferred since its action is considered to be milder). They are also used with **calamine** in milder eczematous skin conditions.

Zinc Paste Bandage, BP 1993
Cotton fabric, plain weave, impregnated with suitable paste containing zinc oxide; requires additional bandaging, 6 m × 7.5 cm = £3.44 (S&N Hlth.—*Viscopaste PB7®* (10%), *excipients: include* cetostearyl alcohol, hydroxybenzoates)

Zinc Paste and Ichthammol Bandage, BP 1993
Cotton fabric, plain weave, impregnated with suitable paste containing zinc oxide and ichthammol; requires additional bandaging, 6 m × 7.5 cm = £3.47 S&N Hlth.—*Ichthopaste®* (6/2%), *excipients: include* cetostearyl alcohol
Uses   see BNF section 13.5

Steripaste® (Mölnlycke)
Cotton fabric, selvedge weave impregnated with paste containing zinc oxide (requires additional bandaging), 6 m × 7.5 cm = £3.24
Excipients   include polysorbate 80

◢ **Medicated stocking**

Zipzoc® (S&N Hlth.)
Sterile rayon stocking impregnated with ointment containing zinc oxide 20%. 4-pouch carton = £12.52; 10-pouch carton = £31.30
Note   Can be used under appropriate compression bandages or hosiery in chronic venous insufficiency

Compression hosiery and garments

Compression (elastic) hosiery is used to treat conditions associated with chronic venous insufficiency, to prevent recurrence of thrombosis, or to reduce the risk of further venous ulceration after treatment with compression bandaging (section A5.8.7). Doppler testing to confirm arterial sufficiency is required before recommending the use of compression hosiery.

Before elastic hosiery can be dispensed, the quantity (single or pair), article (including accessories), and compression class must be specified by the prescriber. There are different compression values for graduated compression hosiery and lymphoedema garments (see table below). All dispensed elastic hosiery articles must state on the packaging that they conform with Drug Tariff technical specification No. 40, for further details see Drug Tariff.

Note Graduated compression tights are .

Compression values for hosiery and lymphoedema garments

Compression class	Compression hosiery (British standard)	Lymphoedema garments (European classification)
Class 1	14–17 mmHg	18–21 mmHg
Class 2	18–24 mmHg	23–32 mmHg
Class 3	25–35 mmHg	34–46 mmHg
Class 4	Not available	49–70 mmHg
Class 4 super	Not available	60–90 mmHg

A5.9.1 Graduated compression hosiery

Class 1 Light Support
Hosiery, compression at ankle 14–17 mmHg, thigh length or below knee with knitted in heel. 1 pair, circular knit (standard), thigh length = £7.61, below knee = £6.95, (made-to-measure), thigh length = £37.79, below knee = £23.64; lightweight elastic net (made-to-measure), thigh length = £20.38, below knee = £15.91

Uses superficial or early varices, varicosis during pregnancy

Class 2 Medium Support
Hosiery, compression at ankle 18–24 mmHg, thigh length or below knee with knitted in heel. 1 pair, circular knit (standard), thigh length = £11.31, below knee = £10.16, (made-to-measure), thigh length = £37.79, below knee = £23.64; net (made-to-measure), thigh length = £20.38, below knee = £15.91; flat bed (made-to-measure, only with closed heel and open toe), thigh length = £37.79, below knee = £23.64

Uses varices of medium severity, ulcer treatment and prophylaxis, mild oedema, varicosis during pregnancy

Class 3 Strong Support
Hosiery, compression at ankle 25–35 mmHg, thigh length or below knee with open or knitted in heel.

1 pair, circular knit (standard), thigh length = £13.40, below knee = £11.52, (made-to-measure) thigh length = £37.79, below knee = £23.64; flat bed (made-to-measure, only with open heel and open toe), thigh length = £37.79, below knee = £23.64

Uses gross varices, post thrombotic venous insufficiency, gross oedema, ulcer treatment and prophylaxis

◀Accessories

In addition to the product listed below, accessories such as application aids for hosiery are available, see Drug Tariff for details

Suspender
Suspender, for thigh stockings = 67p, belt (specification 13), = £5.16, fitted (additional price) = 62p

◀Anklets

Class 2 Medium Support
Anklets, compression 18–24 mmHg, circular knit (standard and made-to-measure), 1 pair = £6.66; flat bed (standard and made-to-measure) = £13.84; net (made-to-measure) = £13.09

Class 3 Strong Support
Anklets, compression 25–35 mmHg, circular knit (standard and made-to-measure), 1 pair = £9.09; flat bed (standard) = £9.29, (made-to-measure) = £13.84

◀Knee caps

Class 2 Medium Support
Kneecaps, compression 18–24 mmHg, circular knit (standard and made-to-measure), 1 pair = £6.66; flat bed (standard and made-to-measure) = £13.84; net (made-to-measure) = £10.87

Class 3 Strong Support
Kneecaps, compression 25–35 mmHg, circular knit (standard and made-to-measure), 1 pair = £8.88; flat bed (standard), (made-to-measure) = £13.84

A5.9.2 Lymphoedema garments

Lymphoedema compression garments are used to maintain limb shape and prevent additional fluid retention. Either flat-bed or circular knitting methods are used in the manufacture of elasticated compression garments. Seamless, circular-knitted garments (in standard sizes) can be used to prevent swelling if the lymphoedema is well controlled and if the limb is in good shape and without skin folds. Flat-knitted garments (usually made-to-measure) with a seam, provide greater rigidity and stiffness to maintain reduction of lymphoedema following treatment with compression bandages.

A standard range of light, medium, or high compression garments are available, as well as low compression (12–16 mmHg) armsleeves, made-to-measure garments up to compression 90 mmHg, and accessories—see Drug Tariff for details.

Note There are different compression values for lymphoedema garments and graduated compression hosiery, see table, p. 61.

Index

Proprietary (trade) names and names of organisms are printed in *italic* type.